Heal Us O Lord

HEAL US O LORD

A Chaplain's Interface with Pain

RABBI SIDNEY GOLDSTEIN, PH.D.

KTAV Publishing

URIM PUBLICATIONS
Jerusalem • New York

To Marilyn,

my life partner, best friend

and anchor of our family

Heal Us O Lord: A Chaplain's Interface with Pain,
by Sidney Goldstein
Copyright © 2018 by Sidney Goldstein
Typeset by Ariel Walden
Printed in Israel
First Edition
ISBN 978-965-524-275-1
KTAV Publishing
527 Empire Boulevard
Brooklyn, NY 11225
www.ktav.com
Urim Publications
P.O. Box 52287
Jerusalem 9152102 Israel
www.UrimPublications.com

Library of Congress Cataloging-in-Publication Data

Names: Goldstein, Sidney, 1935- author.
Title: Heal us O Lord : a chaplain's interface with pain /
Rabbi Sidney Goldstein, Ph.D.
Description: First edition. | Brooklyn, NY: KTAV Publishing ;
Jerusalem : Urim Publications, [2017] | Includes bibliographical
references and index.
Identifiers: LCCN 2017026945 | ISBN 9789655242751 (hardback)
Subjects: LCSH: Goldstein, Sidney, 1935- | Rabbis—United States—
Biography. | Chaplains, Hospital—United States—Biography. |
BISAC: MEDICAL / Caregiving.
Classification: LCC BM755.G643 A3 2017 | DDC 296.6/1—dc23
LC record available at https://lccn.loc.gov/2017026945

PREFACE

THE CHAPLAINCY IS A position which is very emotionally draining. Providing support in a constant and consistent fashion is a burdensome and painful task – although rewarding and gratifying. An important question is, how can the Chaplain achieve a sense of connection with a patient or prisoner? It is often the case that it happens instinctively. No matter how many courses or seminars one takes, the reality is that the Chaplain's combined experiences, upbringing, education, and above all, his home situation will help him forge these significant relationships.

The author has been blessed with a great sense of connectedness with all members of his family. It is this reality which gives him the emotional equilibrium to deal with the many situations that he must face as a Chaplain. The warmth of family life is a significant emotional shield which provides, on the one hand, the protection from being overwhelmed, and on the other hand, gives him the ability to fulfill his duties.

My unstinting love and gratitude are extended to my beloved wife Marilyn with whom I have shared my life. I have always felt, whether in a spoken or unspoken way, the depth of her love and commitment to me and to our wonderful family. Her judgment and intuition have been on target at all times.

Hashem has blessed us with two wonderful daughters,

Amy Tropp and Dr. Julie Fine. They and their devoted husbands Rabbi Mordechai Tropp and Rabbi David Fine have given of themselves, their talents, and their abilities to the welfare of the Jewish community. They have made an enormous difference in countless lives. They and their beautiful families have always been a great source of pride and *nachas* to both my wife and myself. We have been blessed with the intense warmth and love of children, grandchildren, and great-grandchildren. It is this closeness of family which has given me the strength to affect many lives in a most positive way.

To our devoted children Amy and Mordechai, Julie and David; our beloved grandchildren Chaim and Shoshi, Yaakov and Aviva, Chavie and Yoseph, Ephraim, Yitzi, Tova, Aharon, and Moshe Zev; Etan, Chanan, Amiel, and Zachy; our precious great-grandchildren Moshe, Aharon, and Yechezkel; Devorah T., Kayla, Avrumi, and Shayna Rivka; Nechama, Zisi, and Devora L. You have all enriched our lives beyond measure, and to you we pledge our everlasting love and gratitude. May Hashem always shower His beneficence on you throughout your lives.

ACKNOWLEDGEMENTS

I WOULD LIKE TO THANK all those who made this work possible. My gratitude is extended to the countless individuals with whom I have interacted during my years in the Chaplaincy. They include physicians, administrators, prison superintendents, and the heads of various organizations and others who are simply too many to cite. Special mention must be made of the following: the late Ray Alexander who was CEO of the Albert Einstein Medical Center in Philadelphia during the years I served there as Director of Chaplaincy, and the late Dr. Harry Goldberg, Chairman of the Cardiology Department at the same hospital during those years.

My utmost appreciation is extended to Tzvi Mauer of Urim Publications for his deciding to publish my manuscript, and for all his help along the way. I am indebted to my editors Batsheva Pomerantz, Leora Tanenbaum and Michal Alatin for their skillful review, analysis, and refinement of my work. It would not have been the same without their endeavors.

I should also like to thank Dr. Benjamin and Trea Diament, Drs. Paul and Carol Diament, Theodore Diament, Rabbi David and Dr. Julie Fine, Roger and Rebecca Fine, Arnold and Susan Garelick, Howard Klein, Dr. H. Daniel and Adie Roth, William and Ronna Tanenbaum, and Rabbi

Mordechai and Amy Tropp. It is their interest, kindness, and generosity which has made this work possible.

My thanks are extended to the three readers who so graciously read my manuscript and whose comments appear on the back cover. My heartfelt appreciation goes to Nathan Lewin, LLB; Rabbi Dr. Tzvi Schur and Rabbi Dr Norman Strickman for their efforts, comments and validation of my work.

And lastly, thank you to my dear wife Marilyn for reading my manuscript numerous times, for her suggestions, corrections, revisions and especially her patience and support during this entire endeavor.

I T WAS AN INDIAN summer in Philadelphia. The trees near the nursing home exploded with a stunning symphony of red, orange, yellow, and purple leaves. In Rabbi Josh Green's opinion, fall was the fullest time of the year. The brilliant colors, pleasant temperatures, blue skies, and calm winds mingled with a twinge of frost.

The city was full of eclectic and unique neighborhoods, each displaying a quaint, frayed elegance clinging to a glorious past. Philadelphia boasted many "firsts" – first hospital, first savings bank, first university, first public library. If New York was the "Big Apple," Philadelphia was the "Baked Apple" with tangy nuances of years gone by.

The grandmother of Green's wife often referred to an individual who was established and stable as "*gesettled*," an American Yiddishism which she took to mean "settled." Philadelphia was definitely "*gesettled*." It was the hub where the Colonies revolted against the British, bringing to the fore of human history the actualization of liberty, freedom, and democracy – in contrast to other revolutions that brought repression, starvation, murder, dictatorship, and the warping of human creativity. Rabbi Josh Green loved Philadelphia's history and often spoke to patients and staff members about its rich past.

Green was tall and pleasant-looking and walked with a slouch. His wife, Sara, constantly chided him that "he walked like an old man." He would joke with her that among his many deficiencies was a five-o'clock shadow, and that he was constantly fighting the "battle of the bulge."

Green's career had hit an impasse. He had held two good pulpits. However, they were small, and he was at this point not moving up the ladder professionally. He told Sara, in a depressed tone, "My *mazel* has run out."

She replied, "Look, stop feeling sorry for yourself, and go on to Plan B."

"And what might Plan B be?" Green asked cynically.

"Oh, I don't know," Sara said. "You used to like chaplaincy work – why not look into it now?"

Sara was highly intelligent and possessed a keen intuition. She was tall and very attractive with a strong presence. Her voice conveyed a sense of warmth and graciousness. However, she had a temper, which she flashed on occasion. Rushing to prepare for various events and getting ready for the holidays sometimes filled her with anxiety and tension. Her excellent social skills belied her vulnerabilities.

When he held the pulpit, he recognized how difficult a rabbi's life could be. He also began to understand that the wife of a rabbi had a difficult life as well. "What did the *rebbetzin* wear this past Shabbat?" "It was awfully low-cut." "She came in very late last Shabbos." "Her kids run all over the *shul.*" These barbs, tossed at Sara every so often, came back to her through a "friend," and she felt angry and annoyed.

When he was in the pulpit, Green often spared his wife many of the daily difficulties in the congregation. When he was no longer able to tolerate some of the members' misbehaviors, he confided in her. Occasionally, these conversations were helpful since they talked over situations calmly, but sometimes they brought more tension in their wake. Sara would say, "I told you not to tell Goldberg about that." "Ginzburg wasn't the right one to talk to about a raise." "You know you can't trust Cohen about anything." And so on. Then she became infuriated with the members of the synagogue, and sometimes with him! In all, though, he recognized that her advice to him was invariably on target. He always felt that she was the steadying force in his life, and the anchor for love and stability for the entire family.

They met while he was in rabbinical school. He was editor of the Zionist college newspaper of their region and she was a relatively active member of the Zionist youth group to which they both belonged. Sara had been on a year's study trip to Israel. The week after she returned, he asked her to write a report for the paper about her experiences. Actually, he was more interested in her than in the trip. A few days later, he called her to verify the writing assignment and to ask for a date. She agreed. He called her on Thursday for the upcoming Saturday night. He did not know that this was considered an inappropriate move. The social convention of the time called for the man to give a woman almost a week's notice when asking for a date.

When Green rang the bell at Sara's home on Saturday night, her grandmother answered the door. Green asked hesitantly, "Is Sara in?" Sara's grandmother spoke in a very heavy Eastern European accent.

"*Shoower* (sure), come in."

"Sara," the grandmother called, "there is a young man

who is here to see you." Sara walked into the anteroom. She clearly had not been expecting him. She wasn't wearing any make-up. There were still traces of uncamouflaged adolescent acne on her face, and her hair was quite disheveled.

"Josh," she said, "I'm so embarrassed. I thought you meant *next* Saturday night."

Green looked surprised, and mumbled, "I am really sorry. Oh gee," he said in stumbling fashion. "Why then don't we just go out for a walk on the Parkway?" They walked for about an hour and had an ice cream sundae at the local ice cream parlor, and he walked her to her house. They had coffee and cake with her parents. He was struck by their warmth, sociability, and openness. Before he left, he said, "I feel bad about the confusion tonight. Do you think we can see each other next Saturday night?"

"Yes," she said.

After Green left, Sara went into her parents' bedroom. They were in bed reading the newspaper. "So, how did things go?" her father asked.

"Oh, very well," Sara said, "except that there was a mix-up. He meant tonight. I thought he had meant *next* Saturday night."

"I told you," Sara's mother said. "He meant tonight."

"Well, Mom, you were right."

"He looks like a nice fellow," Sara's father said.

"He is," Sara said. "He asked me out for next Saturday night."

"Yeah," her father said, looking a little surprised. "The boy has character."

*

A S THINGS TURNED OUT, Sara was right. Renewed opportunity came for him when he was accepted as Community Chaplain for the Jewish community of Philadelphia and its metropolitan area.

On Mondays he would visit the Blumenfeld Nursing Home. Its impressive entrance was made of marble, which the rabbi thought gave it great dignity. The name "Blumenfeld" was emblazoned across the front. Each time he walked into the lobby, he was met by a portrait of Mr. and Mrs. William Blumenfeld. They had contributed two million dollars toward the building of the home.

Part of the campus included the Malamud Complex, a pleasant group of buildings that served as the residence of the higher-functioning patients with various physical problems, although they were very alert mentally and emotionally. The buildings conveyed an air of warmth, comfort, and security. The flower holders in front of the buildings were filled with geraniums, petunias, impatiens, and pansies. The complex was well-lit, and security guards were always on duty.

The front pathway to the Blumenfeld Nursing Home was lined with well-kept greenery and benches on which the elderly patients would sit with their aides. Often, a patient would sit on the bench, barely aware of his or her surroundings.

It is painful to see life ending in such a dependent and helpless fashion, the rabbi thought. The patients would sometimes sit heads askew, mouths open, staring into space. He felt uncomfortable realizing that many people end their lives in this way. He determined that decline was part of the totality of life's picture. *We often think of life as always reaching upward and onward*, he thought. *Catchwords such as "growth," "development," and "maturity"* had become part of our society's vocabulary, but how about *"debilitation"* and *"weakness"?* What about initials like DNR *(Do Not Resuscitate)* or MI *(medical term for heart attack)?* He smiled to himself as he observed that lately, on TV, this other side of life had gotten through. The rabbi found remarkable that the pert, vivacious actress June Allyson, wife of Dick Powell, the All-American girl, was now advertising products that helped relieve the problems of incontinence. Talk about dissonance! The elderly patients, despite incontinence and dementia, were still deserving of love and care, of being honored as a father or mother. They were still a presence.

Green was sad that so many families were caught in the sandwich of caring for the old and the young – assisting parents who had cared for them but now needed them desperately, and at the same time having to care for their own children.

In Yiddish, there is an expression, an *"ibergekerter velt,"* an upside down world. Young people think they are invulnerable, that the state of life referred to as "youth" is constant, permanent, and everlasting. What if they really could sense the totality of life? Would they think or act differently – would life be more precious? Would they continue to indulge in drugs, binge drinking, and heavy smoking during their teens and college years? Young people came into the nursing home to volunteer, to serve in some way, but can they really sense that the patients represent how everyone ends up in the end? It's hard to understand anything really unless you've experienced it yourself.

Green knew from his experiences in dealing with many families that care at home wasn't feasible in most cases.

Many families simply couldn't afford a full-time companion for their parents. The care was onerous and often involved getting up at all hours. In today's mobile society, the parents could be living in Philadelphia while the children were in Minneapolis. Awful tensions often were created between a couple when an aged and debilitated parent lived with them. Life at all times is worthy of dignity and hope, but how do you provide it to people who are incontinent, no longer lucid, don't respond to a question, and have to be fed? In an imperfect world, the nursing home is the best that can be done.

It was sad, he observed, to see so many of the patients congregate in front of the dining room an hour or so before each meal. They had so little else to do, so they waited. They complained about the food, before, after, and during the meal. At the table, there was very little, if any, discussion. Either they couldn't speak or hear, or they were too depressed to carry on a conversation, or they were too weak to coordinate eating and speaking at the same time. The food was decent, though bland, lacking the spices and salt that most patients could not tolerate. Some patients came into the employee dining room to eat. Either they didn't like the food that was served in the patient dining room, or they came in for a second breakfast or lunch. The staff usually looked the other way. Katie Bramson came regularly and asked various staff people to bring meals to her. She was wheelchair-bound, chunky in build, with a gravelly voice. She had quite a bit of spunk and would often compliment many of the staff by saying, "Sharon, you look sexy today" or "Takisha, the outfit you are wearing is beautiful." She typically wore a pink bathrobe, was always very clean and well-groomed, and knew most of the personnel on a first-name basis.

To anyone who would listen, she recounted the tales of her youth. Her husband had been a prominent men's clothing manufacturer in Philadelphia. They had lived in a prosperous neighborhood. He had died two years ago, and she took care of him until the last days of his life. She and her sister, who lived in Chicago, were extremely close, and they spoke at least once a week. Her son drove a Cadillac, and was a V.P. of an insurance company in affluent Bucks County. Appreciating the compliments and enjoying hearing Katie's life story, the staff bent the rules and brought her breakfast or lunch, which was always the same: a Kaiser roll, a scrambled egg, and coffee. She always made a point of asking for three sugars and a napkin. *Katie Bramson had not succumbed to passivity and helplessness that were such a part of life at the nursing home*, Green thought. The Kaiser roll and the three sugars were symbols of her struggle against the ravages of time and illness. She was in the ring with an 800-pound gorilla and wasn't about to get knocked out easily.

Green often wondered where Katie's resiliency came from. He knew that her family came to America from Vilna, Lithuania when she was eleven years old. Her father had been a tailor and her mother a seamstress. She was three years older than her sister. Katie didn't remember a day she wasn't working. As a youngster, she picked up and delivered orders for her father's clients. During the years of her marriage, she worked in her husband's business. *Perhaps*, Rabbi Green thought, *these early experiences taught her a pleasant aggressiveness that she was able to use now in the waning years of her life, and to survive them better than most.*

*

SOME FAMILIES WOULD VISIT every day. The talk was often limited to questions about the health and condition of the patient. A complaint was voiced about the food, the attendant, the nurse. A son or daughter told the parent about their children and what they were doing, how they were adjusting to school, how they felt about their teachers, how their new marriage was going. Pictures were brought in; an occasional smile appeared on the face of the resident. Sometimes a patient made a remark that the son or daughter found amusing and to the point.

A resident would sometimes ask a visitor, "How old do you think I am?" If the one questioned had a bit of *seichel* (brains), he or she would answer by simply saying, "I don't know." The patient would then respond, "I'm 92."

"Oh my!" the visitor would say in feigned amazement. "I don't believe it! God bless you."

The resident would then respond, "Thank you," exceedingly pleased.

On the whole, the staff appeared cheerful and competent. It was Green's experience that the top echelon – the doctors, nurses, and administrators – were usually capable and well-meaning. The care was inconsistent, however, when it came to the orderlies. Many had little training in this kind of work, or they resented it. Sometimes they were demeaning in how they spoke or dealt with patients. They would refer to a patient by his first name without the patient's or his family's permission. Green thought: *It was discourteous to refer to a man who had had a distinguished professional career, had been married for forty-eight years, and had children, grandchildren, and even great-grandchildren, as Harold, Richard, Bill, or Sam, rather than as Dr., Sir, or Mr.*

Many of the patients were overmedicated and resembled zombies. There was a strong smell of disinfectant throughout the nursing home building. *Life has gotten longer,* Green thought to himself. *But the longer years don't always bring peace and calm.* So many had said to him, "Rabbi, these should be the golden years, but there isn't anything golden about them. They really are very tarnished."

The nursing home was divided into four floors, each containing patients with a different level of consciousness and responsiveness. The top floor disturbed Green the most because it contained those requiring the most care. One could often hear the patients calling someone repeatedly for hours at a time. Sometimes it was a name, "Bill, Bill, Bill." Sometimes it was just a constant sound like "nu, nu, nu." These patients suffered from dementia and were totally dependent on the staff for their care.

Many children of the patients felt guilty about placing their parents in the home. Green understood their feelings. Many would say, "How can we do this to mother or father after all they did for us? We're abandoning them." It was often the child who had invested the most care in the parent who felt the most guilty. Many times the child who lived in California gave advice from afar, stating unequivocally that the parent should be put in the nursing home, and displaying few qualms about it. The cruel paradox was that the ones who gave so much were often plagued by intense guilt feelings while those who contributed so little walked away feeling that they had made the right decision. Often, the pattern followed after the patient entered the nursing home.

The one who cared for the parent the most came to visit the most; those who had been physically and psychologically distant before the parent declined remained distant.

As desolate as the nursing home was, it was even more so for those patients without family at the holidays. Rabbi Green would make a special point of visiting with these patients first. If they were cognizant but too ill to attend services, he would blow the *shofar* for them on Rosh Hashanah or bring them the *lulav* and *etrog* on Sukkot or the matzah on Passover. They were invariably extremely grateful. Green often thought: *To be alone is the most awful thing in the world. You no longer have a sense of belonging, no sense of common shared history with somebody. You were left with no shared mutual moments of calm, frustration, achievement, disillusionment, illness, or recovery.*

Often the nursing home organized theme days such as Mexican Food Day or New Orleans Day. Special menus were created, and even the most compromised would sing at least a few words. The irony was that on New Orleans Day, jazz was played at a high decibel level to accommodate patients who had difficulty hearing – while those whose hearing was strong made faces and complained because the music was too loud. It was good, though, that the home sought to relieve the monotony and melancholia that was so much a part of the place.

Green coordinated special programs, too. The Purim costume programs were particularly popular. The patients were joined by children, grandchildren, and great-grandchildren to share the holiday together. The children would sing and dance, recite nursery rhymes connected with the holiday, and special Purim *hamantaschen* cakes were served. There was usually some response from the patients. They clapped and sang. Green found that music reached even the most afflicted patients. Residents who seemed to be completely out of it managed to sing a few notes of famous Yiddish songs that had been an intrinsic part of their childhood. He found it curious that medical science could not explain how the brain could still conjure up a song even when it wasn't able to do anything else. If an understanding of this paradox could be reached, it might just provide a small part of the answer to the ravages of Alzheimer's, Parkinson's, and other terrible illnesses.

Passover was especially significant at the nursing home. The Bromberg Auditorium was always beautifully decorated. The tables were set with the finest china. Everything glistened. A very expensive Lenox Seder plate was placed in the middle of every table, around which ten people would sit. Families gathered with the parent, since the parent was unable to go home with them for the holiday. It seemed, at least for those two nights of the Seder, that there was some spirit of hope, of freedom from the despair that was so much part of the nursing home. The staff made a special effort to see to it that everything was done right. Passover truly was a special occasion.

Green thought that life, even in severe debilitation, illness, and isolation, was given value when there was continuity because children and grandchildren lent validation to the parent's life. The children's presence effectively declared: "The physical part of your life is waning. Things you did for yourself before are no longer possible. But the historic part, the future beyond yourself, beyond the physical limitation, is still present." And even if the parent couldn't grasp this message, the moment was clearly symbiotic, benefitting both parent and child.

The families came to the tables with their generations. The youngest child recited the classic Four Questions, asking why and how the night of Passover was different from all other nights of the year. Green noticed that some patients responded. It may have just been his imagination in some cases, but even the most debilitated patients said words like "matzah" or "Kiddush," indicating that recognition of Passover remained foundational, even when everything else faded away.

He often wondered how the patients felt at Passover, if indeed they had a sense of awareness at all. They had been heads of families. All the anticipation, work, and effort had been theirs; they had been the ones supervising the Seder reunion with family and friends each year; they had been the center of activity. All the baking, cooking, tension, and anxiety had been theirs to handle. The compliments for the *kneidlach*, the *tzimmes*, and the delicious singular Passover treats; the father sitting at the head of the table, conducting the Seder, assigning responsibilities, explaining the passages of the Haggadah, showing the youngsters the pictures in the Haggadah and what they meant, discussion of politics at mealtime, with emphasis on what was happening to Jews in Israel and throughout the world. All that bore witness to the fact that the holiday penetrated regardless of the patient's deteriorating state.

The home paid for uniformed waiters to serve at the Seder meals, adding a touch of elegance. Many of the family members cried as the Haggadah brought back memories of when they would ask the Four Questions, of coming to the family household with a new bride or husband, of coming with their firstborn and then other children, as the family evolved over time.

The children of the patients would tell Green: "Rabbi, I remember when Mom and Dad had 25 people for the Seder – my brothers and sisters, cousins, aunts and uncles, and now they can hardly feed themselves. What a Seder they made! It was unbelievable. Mom would put up the borscht a month before Passover. Dad would arrange to get the matzah from a special bakery. I would go with him to get the wine and the special Passover cakes and candles. It was something that I looked forward to for a whole year – and now look what's happened."

Green remembered his own Passover as a child, going to *Bubbe* and *Zeide* who lived in the Brownsville section of Brooklyn. His parents piled their mattresses on the roof of a taxi, since his grandparents' apartment wasn't big enough to have a separate bedroom for his parents, and his parents had to place their mattresses in the living room. This was one of the very few times of the year that his parents took a cab. Passover became an excuse for this tiny luxury. His parents had come to America in the mid-1920s. Shortly afterward, the Depression struck. Their psyche was never freed of the trauma of that catastrophic event. Even years later, after they had retired comfortably, they hardly went anywhere and seldom spent money on themselves. When he urged them to take a trip or a cruise, they said that they couldn't because they could not see spending money on themselves. So, for Green as a child, seeing his parents sitting on the mattresses on Passover morning at his grandparents' home symbolized their one extravagance, ironically enough.

The *pièce de résistance* were the goodies – the matzah *kugel*, the sweet Pasternak *kugel* (made with parsnip), the extremely heavy potato *kugel*, which he loved with an almost sensual desire. Who knew of cholesterol then, or triglycerides, or weight control? On the contrary, Green's grandmother always used to use the phrase *"a fetter a gezunter"* – "if you are fat, you are healthy!" Her Passover cooking reflected this attitude. Her honey and sponge cakes were a dream. He often would have at least two pieces with every meal, and as additional snacks throughout the day.

At his grandparents' home there was the very special Haggadah reserved for him every year with a blue cover. Inside were illustrations of the splitting of the Red Sea and the Ten Plagues. Wine had been splattered over the pages over the years. His recital of the *Feer Kashes*, the Four Questions, was anxiously awaited by the family as he stood on his chair and recited the words in the old, familiar singsong chant. He realized he was doing it well when he noticed his father mouthing the words along with him and his mother smiling contentedly and his sister squirmed uncomfortably, waiting for the spotlight to cease shining on her older brother. Green also loved the budding of the trees around Passover time. Many parts of Brooklyn were typically barren, but around Passover, when the few trees in his neighborhood began to bloom, it was as though the borough had been renewed.

All that is gone, he thought. *Bubbe, Zeide, and my father. My sister and I hardly see each other more than twice a year. Mom's living on the West Coast. What did those family Seders mean?*, he wondered. *How did they impact my life? What effect did they have? Like all moments, they were transient – yet captured forever, seared into memory and personality. Maybe that's what's really critical in life. Moments that bottle a shared history of family.*

Where's all of that today? Everybody is so far apart. Neighborhoods seem sterile. Those who grew up in a large Brooklyn tenement knew their "next-*dorikas*" (nextdoor neighbors) very well. Today, people often do not know their neighbors. The physical comforts of the suburbs are often trumped by the sense of isolation that permeates them.

*

GREEN REMEMBERED GROWING UP in Brooklyn. There were hundreds of families on one block. On the days when it was still light after school, the kids went out to play ball on the street. The games were extremely innovative. They had names like punch-ball, stickball, baseball off the wall, flukeball, hit the penny, and boxball. You were considered an all-star if you could punch the ball a distance of two sewers. In flukeball, the goal was to bounce the ball in front of your opponent so that he could not return it. This was achieved by pressing down on the soft Spalding pink ball in such a way that the ball spiraled in unexpected directions. One of Green's great teenage achievements was discovering how to put a reverse spin on the ball so that it became virtually impossible for his opponent to hit it back. He later showed the trick to his nephews. He embellished it by telling them it was actually a magic feat that can be performed only if one whispered an incantation to the ball beseeching it to come back to Uncle Josh. Somehow they believed him!

The kids would go into the street to play ball, or go outside in the spring to eat corn on the cob, wrapped in a napkin, or during the summer to the one locale that then had air-conditioning – the movies. Some of the kids in his neighborhood belonged to the local synagogue. The synagogue sponsored activities and social events and was a very comfortable place.

But today the synagogue, which can provide so much support and a caring community, is virtually non-existent in the lives of many American Jewish youth. Green often reflected that loneliness is the plague of modern society. Today, companionship, support, and comfort are often provided by a professional for a fee. Those who can afford it sometimes see a psychoanalyst three times a week! The Seder today, then, is different from the Seder of yesterday. It is not built on a foundation of mutuality and sharing that is steady throughout the year. It emerges from a year of isolation and loneliness.

Green was struck with how far away everyone was from one another. You can, as the phone company ad used to sing so jubilantly, "reach out and touch someone," but the conversations are often brief and the sense of sharing substantial quality time with a loved one is lacking. We lack these days deep and intense contact with each other. There is no sense of calm, solitude, and peace in our lives. William Wordsworth wrote about two centuries ago: "The world is too much with us." *I wonder*, Josh Green thought, *what he would say now!*

In contrast to the contemporary sense of ennui, the Brooklyn in which Green grew up was a dynamic place. Loneliness was simply not an option. Brooklyn in his time radiated drive, intensity, and ambition. He had many close friends. They were all children of immigrants and they went all-out to make it in America. They would argue with their teachers for every point on their average, as though their entire life depended on their getting a 97 rather than a 95. To them, it did.

The high level of competition was everywhere: A pick-up game in basketball, touch football, and punchball were played with an extreme level of intensity of which New Yorkers, and especially Brooklynites, were capable. Green and his friends discussed every detail of each Brooklyn Dodgers game. They knew the batting averages of all the players, the won and lost records of all the pitchers, and of course, everyone had a take on why the manager had been fired. The talks raged on for weeks when Al Gionfriddo, a journeyman outfielder acquired from Pittsburgh, robbed the great Joe DiMaggio of a home run in Game 6 of the 1947 World Series, helping Brooklyn win the game. The discussions of how he did it went on and on.

When New York Giants outfielder Bobby Thomson had the game-winning home run in the 1950 final playoff game against the Dodgers – "the shot heard 'round the world" (a slight exaggeration) – and the Giants won the pennant, the kids in Brooklyn felt a genuine sense of despair. Some present and former Brooklynites, like Larry King, the famous interviewer, still haven't gotten over it!

Green remembered when Jackie Robinson broke into major league baseball. As a kid, he didn't realize that history was being made. As an adult, the question that sometimes came into his mind was: Why did Robinson break into the majors in Brooklyn and not Philadelphia, Boston, or Chicago, all northern cities? He guessed that those cities at the time would not accept a black player. Brooklyn, with its huge

Jewish population, with a tradition of tolerance and liberalism, would. To prove the point, Ben Chapman, the Phillies' manager in 1947, disgraced himself and his team when he viciously taunted Robinson with miserable racial slurs when Robinson played in Philadelphia.

Brooklyn in the '50s was an opening to America, to its opportunities and its horizons of great plenty. It was an opening that tens of thousands of Jewish kids walked through. In their minds, across that opening was a banner that read, "Don't disappoint your parents."

Many Jewish parents saw in their children an actualization of their own dreams of making it in America – dreams they were unable to accomplish themselves. Most were immigrants, unable to speak English well, and had little formal education. Their lives were filled with struggle, uncertainty, and anxiety. Many had left parents, aunts and uncles, and sisters and brothers in Eastern Europe. As the tides of Hitler's evil rose, their utter helplessness to save their families often cast them into depression and despair. Their kids were their future, their essence, their reason for being.

*

ONE OF THE MOST moving services at the geriatric center was Tisha B'Av, the Ninth Day of Av, the national day of mourning for the Jewish people – the day on which both Temples were destroyed and the Jewish people exiled from their Land. It was very moving to see the patients brought into the synagogue, most by wheelchair. There was a mystical quiet in the synagogue. The sanctuary lights were dimmed. The plaintive lament of the Book of Lamentations penetrated the stillness, and the tone of loss and tragedy permeated the room. The awesome spiritual loss of the Almighty's presence as personified by the destruction of the two Temples was again made real.

In some sense, though, Green thought, *there is hope in Tisha B'Av, even for the residents of the geriatric center. It tells those who have at least some cognition that they are part of an eternal people. Even after so much tragedy and suffering, the Jewish people survive. What awaits them is not only the grave – during life, as after it, they are part of eternity. What a comforting thought this can be for those able to grasp it.*

The Yom Kippur service two months later was filled with pathos. As a young man, the words of the *U'Netaneh Tokef* prayer filled Green with awe. "Who shall live and who shall die," that was a tough one! What *mitzvot* (good deeds) could he perform to help prolong his life? What act of loving-kindness could he do for Mrs. Farber, a neighbor of his, who was 85 and very compromised? Most of the residents of the Blumenfeld Nursing Home, however, did not have to deal with such dilemmas. Death was clearly on the way for most of them, and it was his task to help carry them into the bosom of a loving God.

*

G REEN OFTEN WONDERED HOW the doctors felt about working at the nursing home. The physician's role to cure was, for the most part, absent here. It was a holding operation until the *Malach HaMavet,* the Angel of Death, came. How did it feel to do maintenance, to work with the aged, to know that within a few months or years your patient would be dead? What did it do to one's own sense of vulnerability when one observed people deteriorating every day? Green thought to himself that this must be a very difficult area of medicine to be involved in. What gratifications could there be? Unless . . . there is a feeling of serving another human being, even if there are no prospects for cure. This is medicine *lishmah*, a word often used at the Yeshiva, which referred to "studying Torah for the sake of study itself." Here it was . . . medicine *lishmah* – for the sake of medicine itself. Serving this way is an act of *gemilut chasadim* – an act of loving-kindness. *In all likelihood*, Green thought, *the salaries were decent, although the money was beside the point*. The challenge was to come in every day, to demonstrate compassion and respect, to confront the human element of the profession. Could you show understanding to one with whom you could barely communicate, if at all? Could you show interest in a patient's medical condition even though the disease had progressed and there wasn't much you could do for her? Could you develop a relationship with the families, and call on them for support, when necessary, and see the patient outside of the tunnel of illness as having been once a functioning, capable, vital human being?

His role, too, presented a dilemma. During the first week of his tenure at the home, one of the doctors asked him, "I don't understand, just what is it that you do here?" At the time, he thought to himself: *That makes two of us*. It wasn't the usual congregational situation: the tasks were unstructured; there were no synagogue officers. Visiting the sick was not just a marginal, though important, task: it was the primary task. Talking to many of the patients was often futile since they were unresponsive. At first, the job was depressing, but then he began to challenge himself to relate to patients in an accepting and warm way every day. He began to see the tremendous need that many of the families had for support and understanding. He began to pick up nuances from comments that family members made as to their attitude toward their parents.

It was clear that not all families felt the same way. Some were annoyed that they had to come, and resented visiting the home. Others would visit in a business-like fashion. It was their responsibility, they did it, and that was that, as though that could keep away the emotion and pain of seeing a parent deteriorate and fail. Some would take out their frustrations on the staff and be hypercritical of the conditions. Of course, there were those who came constantly and consistently out of love and devotion.

It made a fascinating study of relationships. Often, if one of the members of the family was wealthier than the others, he would take over, giving instructions to the staff, voicing complaints, and making demands. Old family conflicts that had been dormant for years sometimes came to the fore, especially when there were ethical questions. One case Green remembered particularly well was that of a patient with end-stage heart disease. The doctor had raised the issue of a DNR status with the family. One brother, who lived in Philadelphia close to the father, was very troubled about what to do. His understanding was that everything should be done for his father, and he felt that his father should be resuscitated. The other brother, an attorney living in Washington, D.C., felt that their father should not be resuscitated. The Philadelphian felt that his sibling had cut himself off from the family, visited infrequently, and did not interest himself in their parents' situation – and should not now be voicing an opinion about such a grave matter. The other felt that his brother was too dependent on the father, and that because of this, he could not see the situation with any objectivity, and was wrong in asking that their father be coded. In addition, the patient's wife vacillated as to what to do. They came to Green to discuss the decision.

Green always felt himself very discomfited by these situations. He felt at times that he was playing God. He sought answers to these dilemmas in the *halachah*, Jewish law. The problem was that the *halachah* was often not clear. The way that Green understood it, this was the basic dilemma: Judaism in its infinite respect for human life prohibited any action that actively contributed to an individual's death. On the other hand, Jewish law also had great concern with ending human suffering. As a result of this tension, many questions arise. What about the administration of morphine, which would dull the patient's pain, but because it depresses the respiratory system, can shorten the patient's life?

Green wondered, is one allowed to withhold life support? Distilling the facts from each individual situation, applying the halachah, and, if asked, helping a family to resolve their difficulties was an extremely stressful and intense task. The resolution often left him disoriented for a few days.

Rabbinical school had not prepared him for these dilemmas. The focus had been on the dietary laws and the laws of the Sabbath and holidays. In those years, who knew of a respirator, whether or not to remove it, or when to initiate treatment with it? New technology had brought in its wake many difficult and ethical problems. *Before World War II*, Green often thought, *how much could medicine really do for pa-*

tients? There were no antibiotics, X-rays were primitive, and open heart surgery, and beta blockers were not yet created. What many of the doctors did have, often lacking today, was an aura of warmth and friendship, of being a family friend. The older approach couldn't cure or alleviate pneumonia or arthritis, but it was worth a great deal. *Medicine*, he often thought, *has become too impersonal, too bottom-line conscious.* Maybe that's why there are so many malpractice suits. If the doctor were perceived as a friend, or at least as a source of support, this might not be the case. Today, the doctor is a co-ordinator of lab work and a prescriber of medicine. A good, warm heartfelt talk was often totally beyond his involvement with the patient.

Aside from Passover Seders, many of the families had little connection with religion. However, when it came to end-of-life situations, they wanted the advice of a religious leader. Green chuckled to himself when he remembered that he once walked into a hospital room, introduced himself as Rabbi Green, the hospital chaplain, and the woman in the bed responded, "Oh, I'm not *that* sick."

Most people in these cases wanted to talk, to find stability in the face of suffering and uncertainty. He noticed that often more people sought him out than they did the social worker and psychologist. Those professionals represented the secular disciplines; they were members of the helping professions. In people's minds, he represented what was eternal. He could help cushion the forthcoming loss with a sense of calm and acceptance. It wasn't very easy to maintain a dialogue of assurance while also addressing the family's despair. Sometimes the intensity became so overwhelming that he had to leave the room briefly and return, energized, to continue to help the family deal with the crisis and absorb a sense of calm.

Occasionally, he would chance upon a family talking among themselves in hushed tones about the condition of a parent, about what decisions to make and how to implement them. Sometimes a spouse would stop by in his office and discuss pending funeral plans, even though the patient was not yet terminally ill. He found it very depressing. Everything was planned. The undertaker had carefully enumerated the various provisions, the type of coffin and the price, the skullcaps for the service and their price, the *shiva* benches and how much they would cost, right down to the pending notice in the local newspapers. It was sad, he felt, that everything about death could be labeled – a price set for each item as though one were standing at the checkout counter at a supermarket.

On the other hand, better to know the details, including the prices, in advance. He remembered with great pain how one family in a congregation he had served had not made any provisions. The hasty arrangements were awful. The congregation's plots were full. Another congregation had to be contacted a few hours before the funeral service and a grave was purchased at the last minute. Other things had simply been left undone, unplanned, such as the location of the *shiva* and the provisions for Kaddish. He supposed that the family could not face up to the reality that one day the Malach HaMavet would visit them, just as he visits everyone else.

In a secular world, God is often distant and unreachable. In the nursing home, where suffering is an everyday experience, and life moved in a steady downward graph, faith seemed axiomatic. What gave the suffering meaning? What motivated the families to visit, to care? Was it not an act of faith that prompted family members to reach a deeper relationship than what they ever had achieved before? It all added up to an act of faith, an act that declared to a loved one that his life was and is worthwhile and meaningful, and now as he approached the end, our treatment of him says, "You lived a life of meaning."

*

G REEN OFTEN THOUGHT OF his relationship with his mother. What could he do to add meaning to the last years of her life? He had lost his father ten years ago. His mother, determined to remarry, said she did not want to be an *almanah* (widow). After a false start with one gentleman, she married a very fine man, a widower from California, and she moved there with him. Green saw his mother about once a year, and spoke on the phone to her weekly. But now that he worked at the nursing home, he wanted to do more, to tell her more, to share with her, to make her more a part of his life. Now was the time.

He was ambivalent about his relationship with her. He admired her greatly. She was a dynamic woman with tremendous drive and ambition. She had established a profitable jewelry business, enabling her to put him and his two sisters through college. His father was a lawyer with the federal government. He had a steady job all of his life, but his salary was limited. His mother was essentially the primary economic mainstay. This made family life difficult because she brought the same directness and assertiveness she displayed in business to her role in the family. It was difficult to chal-

34

lenge her, and as a result, he found himself occasionally harboring resentment and hostility toward her. His mother also was a woman who loved learning and culture. She regularly attended lectures and concerts and participated most avidly in the question-and-answer period that followed. Even with her bossiness, he knew that she was completely devoted to him and would do anything she could for him. She had even helped him pay for part of the down payment of his home. Now he felt that before it was too late, it was important to show her how much she meant to him and that he admired her very much.

Yet he felt a wall of unspoken feelings between the two of them. Talking on the phone was not rewarding. The conversations were hurried. He was determined to write at least once a week after she moved to California. At first, his letters were matter-of-fact. He dictated them to his secretary. But over time, he started writing them by hand, and they became more emotionally open. He shared more of his feelings. He knew that his mother appreciated his transformation because once, when she misplaced a letter she received from him, she made a special point of calling him and asking about the contents. This moved him very much.

After someone has children of his own, Green often thought, *he begins to realize what being a parent means. The constant commitment, the concern, the worrying – it's unending.* He was reminded of what Rabbi Isaiah Schwartz at the Yeshiva had once said: "If you don't show your parents *kovod*, respect, after you have children yourself, you are either not much of a person or there is something the matter with you." After he had his own family, he began to recognize the meaning of Rabbi Schwartz's words.

Green understood that honoring parents is not easy. As children, we take their love, presence, and concern for granted. As adolescents, we rebel and often challenge them. As young adults, we begin to make our own way in the world, and often sever ties with them even more. It's all part of the tension that establishing one's autonomy entails. He understood that separating is difficult, and yet it must be accomplished if one is to gain a sense of self. Yet, no matter what, it is important to "honor your father and mother." *It is interesting*, Green thought, *that the Bible does not say, "Love your father and mother.' It says, "Honor your father and mother."* He knew that each home has arguments, tensions, and conflicts. Nevertheless, honoring a parent remains a sacred obligation.

Green remembered wistfully once saying to his parents that he didn't owe them anything, that he resented their staying up until 3:30 a.m. to make sure he was home and safe. He told them that they treated him like a baby. He now remembered how he stayed up himself many nights, spilling into mornings, to wait for his own kids, and how they resented it too, and accused him of babying them. *History repeats itself*, he realized. *Maybe it's only in a parent's final years, when the circle has been closed, when there is a greater sense of acceptance and calm, when the mistakes, foibles, and grudges have receded into the background, maybe it's then and only then that we can see what a parent means.*

Unfortunately, he felt, the mitzvah of honoring parents has been diminished in contemporary America. He had recently discussed the situation with his colleague, Fred Rosenbloom, an old classmate at the Yeshiva, who commented on how much divorce there was in his congregation. Green responded, "It is symptomatic of the general instability of family life and the lack of moral boundaries in America."

"You're probably right, Josh, and you've got to wonder about what's happening to the kids of these divorced parents."

"I'm sure that there is a lot of depression among them," Green said. "You know, Fred, everything is out in the open. I did some reading last summer which really troubled me. All these tell-all confessional books relating the most intimate details of personal family lives – absolutely nothing is held back. And now with the Internet, people really reveal everything."

"I guess people feel they have to vent their feelings, no matter who gets hurt," Rosenbloom said.

"In one of the books I read this past summer," Green said, "a well-known author describes the home she was raised in. It was hell on earth. The father was a violent *meshugener* (crazy person). He continually depreciated his wife and children. She suspected that her brother had AIDS. The mother is described as a neurotic person who was incapable of carrying through on anything."

"I thought that domestic abuse didn't even exist in Jewish homes," Rosenbloom remarked.

"Well," Green said, "that may have been true once, but it isn't anymore. You know, I am talking about the general moral deterioration of American life. I recently read an autobiography by a very well-known journalist who went to all the good schools. He wrote about his late parents' infidelity, the illegitimacy of one of his siblings, and his mother's irresponsible and unrestrained shopping."

"Wow," Rosenbloom joked, "where is HIPPA when you need it?" (The regulations of the Health Insurance Patient

Protection Act which emphasize patient confidentiality.)

"That's cute, Fred," Green responded. "Isn't there something wrong with this picture? Respect for one's parents is being lost in our society. It's the only conclusion I can reach when I read a national magazine – that the daughter of a well-known clergymen, now deceased, writes of the intimate details of his sex life. She also shared with the public her mother's complaints that she was dissatisfied with her physical relationship with her father!"

"I see what you mean," said Rosenbloom. "Everybody just vents and vents until there is no privacy."

"You know, Fred," Green said, "there's no respect for anybody anymore – not for parents, teachers, principals, or clergy."

"Yeah, and it's only getting worse," said Rosenbloom.

*

G REEN ALWAYS WENT OUT of his way to encourage the patients' spouses and children to visit often. He organized an informal therapy group for them. There, he heard many of the frustrations and difficulties they encountered. They expressed great pain that their loved one was suffering, or dismay over how she had deteriorated so rapidly in so short a time. Sometimes Green would hear resentment, too. Al Jacobs, a son of one of the patients, was bitter about his father. He claimed that when he was growing up, his father wasn't very loving and seldom complimented him, and refused to pay for his college education although he could easily have afforded it. Jacobs perceived a great deal of rejection from his father.

38

Green empathized. What should he tell him? How does he help him reconcile how he feels with what is appropriate behavior on the part of a son? Green explained to Jacobs that his visits had value in and of themselves. In all likelihood, he would regret it later if he didn't visit when he could have. And, in the final analysis, visiting his father was a mitzvah – a commandment – unbounded by whether or not the son loved or admired the parent.

This was the most difficult of all the arguments. In a secular world, it was a difficult concept to explain – although in Green's mind, it often made more sense than the oft-cited psychological reasons, many of which did not apply. After all, if a child disliked her parent when she was growing up, and these feelings continued into adulthood and maturity, she wouldn't feel guilty about not visiting the parent often. Sometimes, too, the visits caused so much tension that the child gained no gratification from them. A sacred obligation, however, rendered the child's feelings irrelevant – which perhaps was necessary at the end of a parent's life.

The secular world, Green often thought, *doesn't think in terms of a sacred obligation and commitment. They think in terms of transference, identification, reality testing, ambivalence. All well and good, but these do not encourage fulfilling a mitzvah, doing an act because it conveys holiness and a transcendent commitment.*

Often, Green would be called to talk to a patient in the psychiatric ward, a task he found particularly difficult. Perhaps the patient felt he could work some kind of magic. Often, he worried that the patient would attack him. One, as a matter of fact, tried to; so far, Green was lucky. He wondered how someone with confused thoughts related to him. What did they expect to gain from his visit? Sometimes their statements were so unrealistic that he felt his visit was meaningless.

He found depressed patients extremely challenging. He did his best to be supportive. They would often say, "Rabbi, I keep blaming myself for what happened." They often would castigate themselves for a spouse's death, or for a child's sickness, even though there was no reason for them to believe they held any responsibility. Often, the medication they were taking for their physical conditions weakened them tremendously, leaving them depressed. He pointed out that they held no responsibility for whatever they blamed themselves; they had done what was possible under the circumstances.

The depressed patient, he recognized, wanted validation, wanted to be taken away from the cave in which he found himself. Some knew that there was light outside the cave. They desperately wanted assurance that they could reach the outside. Green felt that his visits provided some calm to these patients, and invariably he felt that they had a positive effect. He could even sense the patient's sighing with a sense of relief when he spoke with them, as though they achieved some catharsis in their emotional state. Despite the self-deprecation and withdrawal, the ruminating and sadness, they wanted to return to that time of their lives when they were happy and well. He assured them that this was possible through therapy and medication. With some, the improvement was in fact minimal; with others, there was significant improvement, and when they would see him after their depression lifted, they would greet him and say, "Rabbi, I'm feeling much better. Thanks for your visit during that very difficult time."

But suicide was a real and ever-present threat. He had

once spoken to a patient in the evening, and the next morning he found out from the nursing staff that the patient had committed suicide. He gyrated with guilt. Had he contributed to the suicide in any way? Had he said the right things? Why didn't he realize that the patient was that sick? Should he have alerted the nurse or psychiatrist? He had difficulty sleeping. Ultimately, he spoke to the staff psychiatrist, who explained that people who are set on committing suicide will find a way – no matter what. The suicide shook him up in other ways, too. He wondered about his own suicidal potential. He had gone through periods of depression, particularly in adolescence. These encounters unnerved him.

His job was all-consuming. People often reached him on the cell phone. The rabbi had moved into hi-tech. Normally, the home phone was an instrument of intrusion into a rabbi's private life. Now it was augmented by the cell phone. It would disturb him at meetings with staff, when he was talking with a patient, when he was planning a lecture, and when he was trying to rest. It got to him at home when he was talking to his wife. Yet the calls were also compliments. People needed him. A nurse wanted him to speak to Mrs. Schwartzberg, a patient in the Malamud Complex; one of the doctors wanted him to speak to Mr. Joseph Weinstein, who was to undergo open heart surgery the next morning. There was great joy in being needed.

Actually, the greatest stress, Green learned, is not having a satisfying expression and outlet for your energies and abilities. He had learned that lesson all too well when he was the rabbi in Bridgeton, New Jersey. The congregation was small and undemanding, and he found it not at all stimulating. It was tough to be in a place where there was no feedback, where the congregants didn't respond to sermons, and where the activity level was low. As he told a colleague, if he would get up in his pajamas at the pulpit on Sabbath morning, the only comment would be that of Mrs. Betty Greenfield, a notorious skinflint, who would tell him, "Rabbi, there's an excellent sale of men's clothing going on at Macy's." Otherwise, there would be no reaction. Even worse was the fact that the congregation was dwindling, and he felt that he was on a sinking ship.

At the nursing home, the situation was different. Here the problem was one of overload and burnout. It was necessary to limit the number of pastoral visits and talks to the patients' families. There was so much to give, and the need was so genuine, and the emotional investment so intense, that he often came home emotionally and physically exhausted. Compassion fatigue, although a new term, was something he fully understood. It was a constantly threatening reality in the work he did.

For the functioning patients at the nursing home, he conducted a morning service – with a *minyan*, a quorum of ten. It was difficult to get the minyan at the assigned time – 7:00 a.m. There were seven regulars, and getting the last three was like pulling teeth. He would ask the *gabbai* – the patient designated as the officer of the congregation – to go to the rooms of three able-bodied residents and call them in. The gabbai's name was Isaac Greenwald. He was a tall, distinguished-looking man who had been one of the original organizers of the minyan. He took a great deal of interest in it and was extremely devoted to maintaining it. He would call "*yahrzeit!*" (the commemoration of the death of a loved one) at the top of his lungs when someone had to recite the memorial prayer for a loved one, and was a *macher*, an influential member, in the best sense of the term. He had about him an air of prosperity and comfort, a reminder that he had been a successful car dealer in Media, Pennsylvania.

His wife Adele was a resident of the Malamud Complex as well. She was a tall, gracious lady, and carried her femininity with great ease. She and her husband were a very attractive couple. They related to each other very well and with great mutual respect. They had two fine sons, Arthur and Joseph, both married. Each had two children whom the Greenwalds doted on as only grandparents can. There was, however, a chronic difficulty which beset the peace and calm of the family. Arthur's wife and Joseph's wife didn't get along. Joseph's wife Evelyn related to the rest of the family in a hostile way. She claimed that Arthur and his family were favored by the Greenwalds, although Rabbi Green felt that this was not the case. She didn't always come along when Joseph went to visit his parents. This was very painful for the entire family.

Mr. Greenwald once asked the rabbi to speak to Evelyn about the situation, and he did. "Listen, Rabbi," Evelyn said. "I know my father-in-law put you up to this. But you know what, I don't care. They're always patronizing us, and they always favor Arthur's kids. Look, everything I have, I earned on my own. I was born into a poor family, did well in college, and went to law school at night while working during the day. Joseph and I have a small law practice and we do all right. Arthur's wife Jane is such a snob. She comes from a wealthy family, and doesn't let you forget it."

Green found it painful that the Greenwalds in their older years had to deal with this kind of tension and hostility.

"When I'm with them I feel very uncomfortable," Evelyn continued, "so as you know I don't come very often."

"Isn't Joseph troubled by your attitude?" Green asked.

"He is," Evelyn said, "but he accepts the situation for what it is. As the kids say, 'It is what it is.'"

"Listen, Evelyn, any time you want to talk, be in touch. I'm here six days a week."

One of the residents of the home was a retired cantor who only came to the minyan if called. Otherwise, he would stay in his apartment. Greenwald was constantly critical of the cantor. There was a running daily battle between them. Greenwald kept challenging the cantor, "Why do you have to wait to be called? We're waiting for you. You should know better, a man of your background and position. You shouldn't require a special invitation." The cantor usually responded that he had to tend to an ailing wife, and that he needed rest early in the morning.

"Yeah, yeah," Greenwald used to say, "I'll bet if there was a fee you'd be here, the first one." This prompted the cantor to refer to Greenwald as an *am ha'aretz*, an ignoramus, and consequently the fight was further enhanced at every turn. *Funny*, thought Green, *here they're coming to pray and they become embroiled in petty differences, infringing on the unifying and uniting theme of the faith.*

It was difficult for some to relate to the other residents in a wholesome way. Green thought: *Maybe this was the way they acted all their lives and now, in the "autumn of their years," they were simply repeating the pattern.* Some had difficult situations with a spouse. This was their way of letting go of some of the pressures they faced once they closed the door of their apartment.

One of the daily attendees at the minyan would sit and give a running commentary about everyone at the minyan and at the residence. The comments were far from charitable or gracious. His name was Ezekiel Abramson. He was a butcher in his younger years, and as the expression goes in the old cowboy movies, "he was one mean, tough hombre." He was deeply resented by the other members of the minyan and who could blame them? Nobody wanted to be called "cheap," "irreligious," "stupid," "ignoramus," or whatever other form of invective Abramson came up with.

As invariably happens in such cases, Abramson's track record wasn't all that great either. His wife complained bitterly about him to all who would listen. His children wanted nothing to do with him, and the home administrators tried to avoid him as much as possible, since he was always complaining about something. He was not especially generous, and never said a positive word to the doctors or nurses with whom he came into contact.

It fell to Green's lot to listen to him, which was not easy. At first he tried to reason with him by showing him a broad picture and pointing out the good qualities of the one Abramson often targeted, Albert Cohen, who was a regular attendee at minyan. He mentioned Cohen's generosity when an appeal was made on the High Holidays. Of course, Abramson always came back with a quick response. "Oh, he's got so much from his years in the black market during the Second World War." When Green pointed out how close, warm, and loving Cohen's relationship was with his wife, Abramson said, "And why not! She was a very wealthy girl when he married her, and he was a *schnorrer* (a beggar) from a very poor home. I knew his family from way back when they lived in the Kensington, a poor neighborhood of the city. They didn't have two nickels to rub together. Millie was the daughter of one of the largest wholesale produce distributors in the city. She was beautiful, too. So, he made out pretty well. You might say he did better than she did, ha, ha!"

When the rabbi praised Jacob Bernstein, another minyan regular, for conducting the services so beautifully, Abramson would respond, "Yes, it was pretty good, but it took much too long, and he mispronounced one of the words in the repetition of the *Amidah*."

When Green praised the dietary staff for preparing a fine meal, Abramson's response was, "The soup was cold." And so it went. Green often thought to himself, *obviously, Abramson is totally ignorant of the song "Accentuate the Positive."*

Often, Green would find himself performing mitzvot when unexpected. A patient would ask him to hold his hand and walk with him to his room. Another would ask him to walk him to religious services. He often thought that the home was a wonderful opportunity to observe the inter-relatedness of life, to show a special level of caring. It was good to be part of a milieu where most everything you did became an emphasized act of loving-kindness. The smile he projected to the patient without family, or to the one whose family visited infrequently, or to the one who was bedridden, resonated through their very being. This was a concept that he hadn't realized when he first joined the staff at the geriatric center. In this environment, even the simplest acts of courtesy and consideration carried great weight. They enhanced the patients' lives immeasurably. Some of the patients became particularly attached to him. They told him, "Rabbi, you're like a breath of fresh air," or, in Yiddish, "*Gut zul dich benchen mit alles gutz*," "God should bless you with everything that is good." As a result, he felt good about what he was doing. This was important validation – the work he was doing was recognized and appreciated! He once asked Mrs. Fanny Silver, a long-time resident, how she was feeling. Her response was, "I wasn't feeling so well until I saw you."

*

PRIOR TO ENTERING THE CHAPLAINCY, Josh Green thought of a rabbinic career in different terms – having a large congregation; officiating at bar mitzvahs, weddings, and funerals; visiting the sick; being actively involved in community affairs and in the political spectrum. The centrality of the role made it appealing. He loved the idea of speaking before large audiences, moralizing, challenging, preaching, educating, being addressed by the title "Rabbi" – as his father once told him, "You're a somebody!" However, the position was 24/7. There was virtually no privacy. Pulpit rabbis' wives had to be involved in congregational affairs, and even their children were targeted for criticism. The loyalty of some of the membership was unstable, and many were always highly critical of whatever he and his family did. As a professor at the seminary once said, "Today's friend is tomorrow's enemy." In short, the position was exhausting, anxiety-provoking, and often put the rabbi on the defensive.

Some congregants were extremely rude. A colleague was once told by the president of his synagogue "to get up on his hind legs and assert himself." Some were cruel. One member of a different synagogue went to the seminary to complain about his rabbi, a friend of Green, without any committee meeting or board conference. That rabbi was in a state of shock and disillusionment for quite a while.

He often heard from colleagues in the pulpit that they felt undervalued and unappreciated – that whatever they did was not enough. Some felt that they were exploited employees, taken for granted. At contract time, some had to go from board member to board member to campaign for a raise or for medical benefits for themselves and their families, as though they were mendicants. On the other hand, some were quite successful. Yet even they were vulnerable. At a conference, he once sat with Rabbi Joshua Borenstein, who had a large and prominent congregation. Some of the colleagues indicated to Rabbi Borenstein that they had heard wonderful things about him from his congregants. He said, "You haven't heard the things they say about me behind my back."

The Chaplaincy had its own unique stresses and challenges. Green had discovered exercise in adolescence as a way to relieve stress and depression. He didn't understand how it worked; he just knew that it did. He exercised "religiously." Aerobic exercise, the treadmill, arm ergometer, swimming, and the stationary bike were his tools in the armamentarium against stress and depression. Still, there were many painful moments.

He once asked a nurse on one of the wards, "How is Mrs. Geraldine Levy in Room 432 today?" and was told, "Rabbi, she expired last night." That word, "expired," had an unrealistic ring to it. It held a kind of never-never land quality, similar to that of "passed away," which is also used to shield others from the realization that one whom they cared for had gone to the Valley of the Shadow of Death. Why couldn't the nurse just have said "died?" "Died" indicated finality. It said that he would never relate to her again. It meant that she and her family would never share moments of joy and sorrow. "Expired" seemed to express a chemical process – objective, clinical, and out of the textbook. "Died," on the other hand, was a one-syllable word hammered into one's consciousness. It said that the person was gone forever. To the rabbi, the term "died" illustrated loss as if with one swift blow: the person was removed from the land of the living and a vacuum had been created forever, never to be filled. The number of the Almighty's souls had diminished for eternity.

He was very moved when staff members came to him for advice and counsel. The administrator of the psychiatric department once walked into his office unexpectedly. She was a single parent rearing two children, and her former husband delayed alimony payments. She was deeply in debt. He suggested that she speak to her creditors personally and that she persuade them to bypass the collection agency. She mentioned that she had lost a child to SIDS, Sudden Infant Death Syndrome. *Some people have no mazel*, he thought. *No luck.* Listening was all he could do.

It was a good feeling to be sought out, to feel that your advice was important. Those who summoned him were from all levels of the occupational spectrum and from all creeds and colors. One of the first counselees was a short, black woman who worked in housekeeping. She was having difficulty with her supervisor. She felt that the supervisor picked on her and was unfair. They spoke regarding her situation. The value of the discussion lay not so much in any suggestions he made but in her ventilating her feeling and emotions about the situation she faced so that she could deal with it from a position of greater emotional security and strength. He was tempted to act like a rescuer, to offer to call the supervisor on her behalf and to intervene. In his early years, he felt that this was the correct approach, that his intervention would somehow help defuse a difficult situation. As he grew more experienced, he saw that intervention was not the best approach. It might alleviate the situation briefly, but on the other hand it might also engender hostility on the part of the supervisor and worsen the employee's situation. The best approach was to strengthen the employee so that she could deal with the situation as wisely as possible.

It was also very meaningful when one of the doctors came in to speak to him about a personal situation. This fostered a collegial relationship. He knew intellectually that doctors had human problems, but the idea that people with such a high level of education and training would have problems similar to all others was dissonant to the rabbi. He remembered vividly how one of the doctors had spoken to him about a family problem. He had been divorced from his wife, who was awarded custody of their child. The wife was indifferent about raising the boy with a Jewish education and preparing him to become a bar mitzvah. The doctor was concerned and asked the rabbi what could be done. Green suggested that the doctor speak to his former father-in-law, a doctor at the home with whom he was on good terms. It was a decent approach, which the doctor in his distress did not think of. As similar circumstances occurred, Green felt himself increasingly an integral member of the staff. His relationships touched all employees and professional staff on all levels.

Sometimes patients grappled with theological issues regarding suffering. He had been asked by a wife to go see her husband. "He's having a great deal of distress, Rabbi. He's wondering about the meaning of his life, and he's quite depressed. He hardly speaks to me. He was always a very thoughtful man. He loved reading and he did very well in his profession. Maybe if you went in to speak to him, he would feel better and would share some of his thoughts with you."

Green walked into the patient's room and spoke with him for a few moments. It was everyday chatter about family and work. Then there was a pause, and he asked, "What did I do to deserve this suffering?" Sometimes the patient inquired, "Why did this happen to me? I was always a good person. I helped others to the extent of my ability. I was a good husband and father."

In the Jobian response, suffering is understood as "God's ways," which are unfathomable. No one can really understand them; they are not necessarily correlated to one's behavior and actions. What else could you really tell the patient? To correlate the patient's suffering with some misdeed would clearly be counterproductive to any recovery that the patient might achieve. In addition, as in the classic case of Job, it clearly was true that the majority of people lived decent, honorable lives and were devoted spouses and parents. The suffering was incomprehensible on that basis. God's plan was difficult to understand. What Green found significant was that all these questions were asked within the structure of belief. "Why did God do this to me?" is an axiomatic acceptance of God's presence by trying to fathom their reality. It was not an unhealthy response under the circumstances.

But Green chuckled as he recalled how quickly deep questions could segue to scatological humor. With one patient, Green waited for him to express his feelings of vulnerability, of existential angst, doubt, and questioning. Instead, the man turned to him and said, "Rabbi, could you please bring over the bedpan?"

Green's sermons, by necessity, were poignant. Residents of the nursing home wanted their last years to be meaningful. To those who could understand and respond, he spoke in terms of the value of these years: to strengthen bonds with children and grandchildren. To residents of the apartment complex, most of whom were lucid, he urged them not to exclude themselves from their families' lives, but rather to strengthen efforts to become an even greater part of them. Often, he told them, "We don't see the impact that we can have on the lives of our grandchildren. They are, in fact, in many ways removed from us, but still that doesn't mean that we can't interact with them. For instance, I know we are concerned that our grandchildren remain Jews. Well, those of us who can, should make them 'an offer they can't refuse.' What if we were to offer them a trip to Israel as a high school graduation present, or at least offer to pay for part of a trip to Israel? Clearly, we would be making a very substantial statement."

It was vital to maintain a cheerful attitude so that the services would be a source of encouragement to these patients and they would be eager to come to them. One of the great personal challenges to him was to project an image of hope and cheerfulness in a difficult situation, to look into this "vale of tears" and give it validation, to demonstrate that even decline had value and meaning. It wasn't, as the sportswriters say about a team that has lost all hope for winning a championship, "playing out the string until the end of the season." He felt it was his task to demonstrate to them that this part of their lives had meaning in and of itself. That's why it was important to enter a patient's room with a pleasant demeanor, or speak to a patient with understanding. He felt his role had an existential and transcendent purpose. He was often asked by colleagues, "Josh, how can you take that, day in and day out? I think that would overwhelm me." He understood what they meant and probably would have thought the same way six years earlier.

Now he saw the situation quite differently. The task was enormously challenging. It involved developing special sensitivities and relationships, understanding ethical questions, an appreciation of seizing the moment because what lay ahead was frightening. It urged him to strengthen his own life in light of what he often jokingly referred to as the "coming attractions." It often tore the veil of illusion from life, an illusion that everyone sought to maintain in the desperate battle against vulnerability and mortality. To fight that battle, many sought different battlegrounds – gambling, alcohol, illicit sexual impulses, workaholism; all were expressions of this drive to outwit and vanquish mortality. He faced that reality every day. Sometimes it became overwhelming or close to it, but by the same token it also underlined the value of what he was doing.

In an effort to personalize the patients, the nursing home placed on the door of each room a brief biographical sketch. Charles Levy in Room 521 had been a cab driver and was a bachelor. Mrs. Marion Brenner in Room 560 had graduated from Juilliard in New York City and was an accomplished concert pianist. She had married a well-known impresario, Jonathan Shick, and had one son, William, who was a professor of medicine at Case Western Reserve University. Robert Cohn in Room 240 had been a law professor at George Washington University in Washington, D.C., and had been a well-known authority in constitutional law. He was married and had three children. His wife, a successful attorney, visited him very often. Green found these biographies fascinating because they rounded the circle of the lives that he saw only in their deteriorated state. Now he could envision what once was.

Green often used these biographies as a jumping-off point for his discussions with the families and the patients. The contrast with what was in the past and the reality of the present was extreme. But, as it says in Ecclesiastes: "Everything has its season, and there is a time for everything under the heavens." The present at the Blumenfeld Nursing Home was a time for support, compassion, and caring, and it was his responsibility to provide these things.

William Weiner was a resident of Room 522 in the complex. He was a warm and vivacious person. Whenever Green would come in, he would greet him graciously, "Rabbi, please come in, I'm so glad to see you." Weiner had been a proprietor of a small fruit and produce store in the Mayfair section of the city, a predominantly middle-class neighborhood with most of the residents living in walkups or apartment houses. Weiner ran the business with his wife, Belle, an energetic and alert woman and one of the most faithful visitors at the complex. She came every morning, made certain that all of Weiner's clothes were in good shape, that he ate his meals, and his room was clean. She would also help the other patients. She fed those who needed to be fed, wheeled those who wanted to go into the activity area, and looked after those who needed various items. Since there was a nursing shortage, the staff always looked forward to her coming. From discussions with their two sons and their families, Green learned something more about William Weiner's background. He had come to America from Galicia as a boy of 18 with his mother. His father had come to America earlier but had become stranded by World War I, and Weiner didn't see his father for nine years. Weiner got various jobs when he immigrated, and then entered the jewelry business as an engraver. He did very well in that line of work until his eyesight began to falter.

Weiner married Belle, who came from the same town in Galicia as he did. They then moved to Carteret, New Jersey, where Belle's brother owned a large grocery store and needed someone to help him out. Weiner liked to chat, and he told Green in one of their discussions, "Rabbi, that's a very tough business. It's day and night. We were enslaved. My mother lived with us, so she took care of the kids while Belle and I helped her brother in the store. Shortly after we started there, her brother got sick with a severe heart attack and was told by his doctors that he had to spend the winters in Florida. The burden of that large store fell on Belle and myself. We would come into the store at six o'clock in the morning and didn't leave until eight thirty at night. The work was backbreaking."

"Did you have any help?" Green asked.

"We had one clerk, but he wasn't particularly reliable or trustworthy. The whole business fell on Belle and me to run. In various ways her brother, Bob, would hint that he would make me a partner, but it never came about. Most of the business was owned by his father-in-law, so I'm not sure that Bob could have made the offer in the first place."

"How was life, generally, in a small town?" Green asked.

"Oh, it was very pleasant," Weiner said. "We had a very nice circle of friends. I became active in the volunteer fire department and the shul. We lived in a big house which was very comfortable, but you know, Rabbi, the life there is limited. We wanted the boys to have more of a Jewish education. So when the partnership with Bob didn't work out, we decided to move to Philadelphia."

"And what did you do here?" Green asked

"We opened the produce store in Mayfair."

"How was business?"

"It was pretty good. The hours were long and the work was backbreaking. I had to carry large crates of fruits and vegetables. We delivered to people's homes, so that meant carrying very substantial loads on my shoulders for three or more flights of stairs. Fortunately, my health held up enough to put the boys through school."

"Well, you certainly have a lot to be proud of. The boys are very fine and accomplished and very devoted."

"Thank you, Rabbi. Yes, Belle and I are very proud of them and they certainly show their devotion to us in many ways."

"They sure do," Green agreed. "It's not often you see sons coming two and three times a week to visit with a parent in the home."

"Yes, I know," Weiner said. "I often tell Belle that we may not be rich in money, but we are rich in our children."

"That certainly is the greatest asset," Green said. "*Nachas* from children is a very big thing."

"The biggest thing! Rabbi. I'll tell you, a few dollars more or less doesn't mean all that much. If you can look at your children and say that they are following in your ways, and then some, then you can say your life has been fulfilled." Tears gently dropped from his eyes.

"You know, during the course of my working years, I wasn't able to keep the Sabbath. Once I retired, though, I was determined to do so. Belle and I decided that no matter what, we would give the boys a Jewish education. I'm glad that we did and today they are observant young men and raising their children that way."

Green saw that Weiner had created his own personality, which was quite remarkable. To be without a father for nine crucial years, and yet to have remained pleasant and warm, was a very substantial accomplishment.

What experiences did Weiner have during the course of his lifetime that made him the kind, generous, and gracious person that he obviously was? Was his mother a kind and gentle woman who raised him that way, despite his father's absence? Were there other members of the family who gave him the necessary support?

Green thought so much emphasis is placed in contemporary society on early childhood experiences. How much do we really know about character development? Is there just a randomness about human life that influences everything and is really beyond analysis and comprehension? Was it the society in which Weiner grew up that preached a sense of responsibility, hard work, respect for parents, and a strong moral code? Did this help to form his fine character?

Room 438 was occupied by Howard Grossman, who had been an attorney for the Legal Aid Society. He was a man of medium height with a kindly face and a very light complexion. He was flattered that the rabbi came in to see him regularly. Green thought to himself: *This older generation was raised with a sense of respect for a rabbi, something that many young people today do not demonstrate. They are so full of themselves and their own material success and achievements that the spiritual side of life, and those who represent it, are not valued.*

"Come in, Rabbi," Grossman said, rising from his chair. "Please sit down."

"Oh, thanks, Mr. Grossman," Green said courteously, "you don't have to stand for me. How are you doing today, Mr. Grossman?"

"Oh, pretty good, Rabbi," Grossman said with something of a sigh. Grossman appeared to be somewhat depressed all the time, as though some cloud of melancholia hovered over him. He also seemed anxious, although this did not affect his conversations or his relationships with the other residents. He was well-liked by them and related to them well.

"Rabbi," he asked Green, "how long have you been in the rabbinate?"

"It's fifteen years now, Mr. Grossman. Why do you ask?"

"Well, you look quite young to be a rabbi."

"Thank you," Green said. "You made my day."

Grossman smiled, "No, really," he said, "you look quite young. Do you have a family?"

"Oh, yes," Green said, nodding vigorously. "My wife and I have been blessed with two lovely daughters."

"Oh, that's nice. What do they say, a son is a son till he takes a wife. A daughter's a daughter for life, and you're blessed with two. Please tell me more about them."

"Well," Green said, "the older one Lisa has always been

very competitive. I remember when she was very little, playing a kids' game with her called Candyland and she lost. She became infuriated and carried on something awful. She was active in her youth group and set her sights on becoming president. Needless to say, she became president. Then she became president of the student body at her school. Actually, her favorite role – whether at school or at the organizations she belonged to – was that of President."

"You've really got a pretty ambitious kid there, maybe one day she will grow up to be President of the United States."

"I'll tell you, Mr. Grossman," Green chuckled, "I wouldn't want her to aspire to that job, she might just get it. In truth, Mr. Grossman, it is not only her competitiveness that won her these positions, it is her kindness, consideration, and compassion for others as well as her trustworthiness that even her young peers recognize."

"How about your younger one?" Grossman asked.

"Our younger one, Rachel, is a budding psychologist. From very early childhood she would analyze motives of both kids and adults and tell them what they were – she was usually right. My wife and I tried to dissuade her from doing this and told her that people don't appreciate having a mirror held up to their psyches and that she best wait until she became a psychologist. Of course, she continued doing her own thing. All in all, though, she is a very colorful kid and is always lots of fun."

"Rabbi, it sounds like you and your wife are enjoying both your kids."

"Mr. Grossman, that's a wonderful way of putting it. Oh, that's enough about me. Tell me something about yourself."

"Well, Rabbi, I was born in Lithuania in a city called Lida.

It was a very religious town. The well-known Rabbi Daniel Levinson was the rabbi of the town. As a matter of fact, he taught Talmud at the Maimonides Rabbinical Seminary in New York City."

"Yes," Green said. "He was my teacher for a year."

"Really, that's interesting," Grossman said. "It's too bad that my family lost touch with him once we came to America. At any rate, when my family came to America, they settled in Albany, Georgia."

"Albany, Georgia," Green responded in a surprised tone. "What brought your folks to a town in the Deep South?"

"Well, you know, Rabbi, it was business. Pop, *alav hasha-lom*, of blessed memory, saw an opportunity to go into the dry goods business down there and he took it. His brother had already established a business there and had urged him to join with him. America was new and strange, big city life was overwhelming, so he joined his brother."

"And how did you like living down there?"

"It was alright. Actually, it was a pretty good place to, as they say in Yiddish, '*oistzigreening*,' to get over being a green-horn. We could speak Yiddish only at home. Outside we had to speak English. I came to America when I was fourteen. I went straight into high school."

"And how did you do?"

"Oh, pretty well. The teachers were very demanding. I still remember my Latin and English teachers. They were rough, and the discipline, my goodness, the discipline was tight. You couldn't get away with anything, not like today where anything goes."

"Did you encounter any anti-Semitism there?"

"No, I can't say that I did. I was the only Jewish boy in the class, but I was always treated fairly and, you know the way it is in a small town, you're sort of one big family. My folks had a good reputation, and they did well. As far as I could tell, the Jewish community had about fifty families, and we were treated very decently and occupied a respected place in the town. But I wanted to leave Albany. It was OK, but it was too isolated," Grossman said, taking off his glasses, breathing on them, and cleaning them with a tissue. "So I went on to college at NYU."

"You might say," Green said jokingly, "that the Old South prepared a Jewish boy from Eastern Europe for life in the North."

"Yes, that's right," Grossman chuckled.

"Did you like New York, Mr. Grossman? That was quite a switch after Albany, Georgia."

"You bet it was, Rabbi. New York was fine. In those days, it was a different city. You could ride the subway at 2:00 a.m., and nobody would bother you. The cultural life was, of course, wonderful and varied. The intensity of life, of striving, of trying to 'make it in America' was everywhere. You couldn't avoid it. It was really a very special place at that time. It still is, although the quality of life has deteriorated."

"And what did you do afterward?" Green asked, pushing his yarmulke down on his head a little.

"Well, after I graduated from NYU, I went on to their law school."

"That was a very fine achievement," Green said.

"Yes, thank you, I worked hard. I always enjoyed learning and studying and was able to apply myself."

"And did you practice law?" Green asked, glancing at the name tag above Grossman's bed.

"I took a job with the Legal Aid Society. It was Depression time; jobs were very hard to get. This opportunity came up. The salary was decent, nothing to get excited about, but the job was a stable one, and I stayed with them for forty years."

"You're what they call a loyal employee," Green said, rubbing his chin.

"Yes, I was," Grossman said, with a pleasant smile of affirmation. "I gave it my best shot, I'll tell you. It was good helping poor people and advising them as to their legal rights. You know, we were one of the few agencies that looked out for the indigent and tried to get them a break in the justice system. I felt good about doing that. To help a millionaire save money on his taxes or prosecute some Mafia type didn't appeal to me. This was a good way to use my legal education to help others, and that meant a lot to me. I often got letters of thanks from clients, and that was a very good feeling. I felt that I was one of the few resources they had. I've got no complaints. I was treated well, and I liked what I was doing."

"Do you have a family, Mr. Grossman?"

"Oh, yes. My late wife and I have a son and a daughter. My son, whose name is David, is finishing law school this year, and my daughter, Rebecca, is in her third year of college here at the University of Pennsylvania. They're really good kids. My son finished NYU *magna cum laude* and is now at their law school," Grossman said, beaming. "He's a really smart boy and has won all kinds of prizes. As a matter of fact, he was a Fulbright Scholar. He speaks very well publicly and is a very fine looking kid. He's going with a very nice girl, who comes from a lovely family." Grossman got up and pointed to a picture of a pleasant-looking young man on his night table.

"He is a very nice-looking fellow," Green said, "and I see that you're very proud of him."

"Thank you, Rabbi, I sure am."

"And your daughter, Mr. Grossman, how about her?"

"She's studying English Lit." Grossman's eyes sparkled when he said this. "She's very bright and has done some really good writing. She had some of her work published in *The Daily Pennsylvanian*, and has written two short plays which were performed at the camp where she was a Dramatics counselor. This is her picture, Rabbi."

Green looked at the photo of a very lovely, smiling blond-haired girl.

"I pray that they should both have a lot of *mazel* in their lives. I lost my wife three years ago, after being married for thirty-five years. They're really all I have," Grossman said in a depressed tone.

"Well, God should be good to them," Green said, "and you should have *nachas*." Green thought, as he left the room, *Grossman is so extremely proud of his kids. They're probably filling the gaps that he perceives his life to have had. Well, God bless him. I guess he tells many people of his kids' achievements, and that's not an easy burden for kids to carry. They probably are very embarrassed by it. But you know what, it's not terrible! I'm sure that he was a decent and considerate father, all his life, so now it's payback time for him! I hope that his kids handle the situation well, for everyone's sake.*

The occupant of Room 623 in the Malamud building was Ellen Rosenblatt. She was a gruff person and, at first, Green was put off by her manner. At the beginning of their relationship, she greeted him coldly and he found that it was difficult getting through to her. After a while, though, she began responding in a more kindly manner and he found that she was in fact easier to relate to than he thought at first. Her story was quite moving.

"Mrs. Rosenblatt," Green said, knocking on her door. "It's Rabbi Green."

"Rabbi, come in," she answered plainly.

He entered a nicely decorated room. Mrs. Rosenblatt's grandchildren had sent her cards and flowers for her birthday which took up the entire window sill and the top of her night table. She was sitting in her bathrobe decorated with flowers of all different colors. This all added a sense of cheerfulness and light to an otherwise standard room.

"Mrs. Rosenblatt, that's a beautiful bathrobe you've got on. Is it new?"

"Yes, it's a birthday present from my two grandchildren."

"You know, Mrs. Rosenblatt, that's a coat of many colors."

"Yes, that's right," Mrs. Rosenblatt said, smiling. "It means a great deal to me since they are the only family I have left. I lost my only child, a daughter, ten years ago and my husband of forty years died two years ago. You know, Rabbi, I've had a difficult life, but I'm not complaining. God's been good to me in many ways, too."

"Tell me a little about your life, Mrs. Rosenblatt," Green said in a supportive tone.

"My father came from Bridgeport, Connecticut. He learned of an opportunity here in the window cleaning business. We came to Philadelphia when I was nine and my two brothers were six and three."

"How did your father do, once he came here?"

"At first he did quite well. He got some very big accounts. We lived in a nice house over in the Mount Airy section of the city, which in those days was one of the better neighborhoods. My two brothers and I always wore fine clothes and never lacked for anything. One day my father got a call from one of his workers, who told him that he couldn't come to work that day. My father wasn't feeling well, but he went in anyway in place of the worker. That night, he complained of chest pains. In the morning he was dead; he died in his sleep at the age of thirty-eight," Mrs. Rosenblatt said tearfully. "My mother was beside herself. I guess from the shock and suddenness of what happened, she took ill herself and died a year later."

"And you were left with two younger brothers, alone in the world?"

"Yes, that's what happened. Except that we were lucky. My father's sister had been married for ten years and was childless. When this tragedy happened, she said that God had now given her the opportunity to have a family of her own. She did not want us to be put in a state institution, so she and my uncle took us in. My aunt and uncle received support from the state to maintain us."

"What were your aunt and uncle's names?" Green asked.

"Aunt Esther and Uncle Nachman."

"How did they treat you?"

"Oh, they treated us very well. My aunt was really like a mother to us. She cared for us all in a very loving and kindly way. My uncle was a little, as they say in Yiddish, *'prust,'* boorish. He was basically a good-natured person, but he would curse a lot and was not refined. I will say this, though: he never mistreated us in any way. It's just that he was a common person and really didn't know how to deal with situations too well."

"When did you start working?"

"Well, I got a job in a department store at the age of six-teen and earned pretty good money for a girl my age, and for that time. I must say I was quite a girl. I took a great deal of pride in what I did and was well-liked by everyone in the store. From the stock room, I was promoted to be a salesgirl in women's wear. I really liked that job a lot. We dealt with a very fine clientele and I met some very cultured and well-to-do people. They would always ask to see Ellen when they came into the store."

"And how did you meet your husband, Mrs. Rosenblatt?" Green asked quietly.

"He was a buyer for one of the large chains and would come into the store frequently. We met over the counter, you might say," she chuckled. "We dated for a year and we married in 1935."

"That was right during the height of the Depression, wasn't it?"

"Yes, a year after we were married, my husband lost his job. Things were so bad! But soon afterward he got a job with the federal government in the post office. He was with them for forty years before he retired in 1977."

"And do you have other family, Mrs. Rosenblatt?"

"Yes, my two brothers are still alive. One lives in Florida with a son, and the other in California with a daughter. I write to them fairly often but don't see them much."

"And you said that you had a daughter?"

"Yes, we had one beautiful daughter," Mrs. Rosenblatt said, dabbing her eyes with her handkerchief. "She died of cancer when she was thirty-five. She left two children, a son and a daughter. I had to go on. I had to help their father raise the two children. What else could I do?" she said, crying softly.

"How are the kids now?"

"They turned out fine. They're both married. They married Jewish kids, too. They both live near here. We're very close, as you can see." Mrs. Rosenblatt pointed to the window sill.

"Mrs. Rosenblatt, you really are a heroic woman. God bless you with strength and stamina to continue to be strong."

"Rabbi, I really appreciate your coming in to see me. God has given me the strength, up to now. I pray that He will continue to do so in the future. Rabbi, you're young, your perception of life is different from mine. I'm sure yours is flavored with optimism and promise, and that's the way it should be. Mine is leavened with sorrow, but also with acceptance. I do believe in God, and whatever God has in mind for me I accept fully; I'm just not ready for Him to take me yet. Before going to sleep, I tell my late husband, 'Don't worry, I'm coming to greet you, but not so soon!'" A melancholy smile enveloped her pretty face.

The resident in Room 530 was Bill Danzig. A construction worker all his life, he was a big, hearty man with red cheeks and a substantial paunch that he jokingly patted and referred to as his "corporation." His appetite at mealtime was notorious. Invariably, he had double and often triple portions. Behind his back, many of the residents would refer to him as a *chazir*, a pig. Green found Danzig to be a very affable sort who helped out whenever he could. From transporting prayer books, to wheeling patients into services, to bringing a patient the Sabbath candles, Danzig did it. The rabbi visited Danzig quite often, finding him very cheerful, and this provided a pleasant change of pace from some of the melancholy aspects of his routine.

"Bill, are you there?" Green said, knocking at the door of 530.

"C'mon in," Danzig said in a booming voice. "Sit down over here," pointing to a chair while removing a blanket which he had placed on it. "Rabbi, I'm sure glad you came in. I was just reading an article in *The Jewish Weekly Press*, and there's something I wanted to ask you. The writer here says that most of the Jewish people living in Israel are not religious. Is this so?"

"Oh yes, Bill," Green said. "I guess at least 75 percent are not."

"Is that so," Danzig said, "I'm really surprised."

"Well, you know, Bill, Israel was founded primarily by secular Zionists. They were for the most part the pioneers of the State. Not that there weren't religious Zionists who played a role, but it was primarily secular Zionists who formed the State."

"You mean, Rabbi, that those who came to Israel in the early years were *goyim*?" Danzig asked in his usual gruff manner.

"Bill," Green said with a smile, "that's a good one. They were not gentiles, of course, just that in most cases they were people looking to express their Jewishness in what they felt would be a different and more dynamic way. They saw the practice of Judaism as being part of what they called '*galut*,' which meant being a stranger in the land that you were living in, suffering persecution, with no economic opportunity, especially in Eastern Europe. They felt that they had to leave all that and renew Jewish life in the ancient homeland, in what was then called Palestine."

"And how about the religious people?" Danzig asked.

"Some of them joined in, but many were opposed to the building of a Jewish State through human means. They felt that it should come through supernatural means, through the coming of the Messiah. As a result, that's why most of the Jews in Israel today aren't religious."

"Do you think this might change, Rabbi?"

"I don't think that it will happen on some sort of mass scale, but perhaps on an individual basis. I think that many in Israel are looking for an alternative to a secular lifestyle, which is not satisfying to many because it doesn't project a transcendent set of values. They're looking for something to be a source of stability and hope."

"You mean like the rudder on a ship?"

"Yeah, that's a good analogy, Bill." Green was pleased with Danzig's gruff intelligence. "Anyway, Bill, enough about Israel. Tell me about you. Where you're from, your family, your job. You've never really given me the lowdown."

"Well, Rabbi, what can I tell you? I was a construction worker for many years with the Cunningham Construction Company in Philadelphia. I had a good job. I made very good money and lived very well."

"Did you work on many big jobs?"

"Oh yeah, we built the Washington Center in Center City and the Hamilton Bank Building in the King of Prussia area. It was really a major league corporation in those years. At one time we employed over a thousand people."

"That really sounds like a large outfit," Green said, smoothing his jacket.

"At one time we were the second largest in the North-east," Danzig said. "I was a Union Shop Steward, and was a real big shot."

"Were they a good company to work for?"

"Oh yeah," Danzig said. "They paid well and they had a very good benefits package. The only thing was the work had many ups and downs, depending on the real estate market. Some years it was great and other years it was lousy," Danzig said, pointing his thumb downwards. "But I did very well."

"Bill, were you ever married? Do you have a family?"

"No, I never did marry," Danzig said. "I couldn't find Ms. Wonderful, although I never lacked for female companion-ship, if you know what I mean," Danzig said with a wink.

"Yes, I do," Green said.

"I always treated the ladies well – real well. You name it! I took them to Las Vegas, Atlantic City, Miami, Bermuda. I had a good time, a real good time, Rabbi," Danzig said with the braggadocio that made him so colorful and so scorned.

"Did you live alone?"

"No, I lived with Mom until she died about ten years ago. She was a wonderful woman, so kind and gracious and real religious, too. She always lit candles Friday night and davened every day. I still remember her saying the prayer '*Gut Fun Avraham*' ('God of Abraham,' Yiddish prayer) at the end of Shabbos." Danzig said, wiping his eyes. "And so charitable. There was a *pushka* on the window sill in the kitchen, and every evening she would put in a few cents and, believe me, Rabbi, for many years she didn't have much, not much at all."

"She sounds like a real traditional type of Jewish woman from, as they say, 'the old school,'" Green said in a kindly way.

"She sure was, Rabbi, they don't make them that way anymore."

"And what brought you here to this geriatric center?"

"I have a cousin here who is well-connected. He is very well-off, '*ungeshtupt*,' '*mucho dinero*' – you know what I mean. He was able to use his influence to get me in."

"Rabbi, I didn't feel like cooking for myself anymore, and living alone wasn't satisfying, so I spoke to my cousin. I knew that he was active here, and he suggested that I apply, and because of his influence I was accepted. It's fine and I'm pleased to be here. They serve three meals a day, and they have social activities. I'm busy and active, and quite satisfied."

"Well, Bill, I certainly appreciate your help at our religious activities."

"Please don't thank me. It's my pleasure."

Green thought to himself, as he left Danzig's room: *It's good to have a fellow like Danzig. He is helpful, and in his own brusque way understands what loyalty means.*

Dr. Sonja Borislov was the resident in Room 232. She had received her medical diploma from Moscow University in pediatrics. When the Soviet Union became unstable for Jews, she left with her husband and two children for America. Green always liked speaking to her. She was highly intelligent and cultured, and was always interested in discussing Jewish religion and culture. She looked like the stereotypical Russian babushka – short, squat, with a round, pleasant face, and with two gold teeth right in the middle of her mouth. She smiled frequently, so that her gold teeth often reflected the light in the nursing home. Some of the residents referred to her fondly as the "*shtikel gold*," a piece of gold. She spoke with a heavy Russian accent, and would often weave in a few Russian phrases in her speech. She was well-liked by the administration, residents, and staff. She also served as a Russian interpreter when the need arose.

Green knocked on the door of her room tentatively, unsure if she was in. "Sonja, Dr. Borislov," Green called, "it's Rabbi Green."

"Yes," she replied from the bathroom in the room. "I'll be right out. Just please wait."

She came out shortly and said, "Rabbi," extending the "a" with her Russian accent. "I'm so glad to see you."

"Same here, Sonja," Green said with affirmation. "It's always a pleasure to visit with you."

"Rabbi, you know, I really enjoyed the services last Shabbat. When I was growing up in the Soviet Union, I didn't have a chance to be exposed to any Jewish education. The regime just didn't permit it. We were taught that religion was false, that Judaism was a superstition, and that Zionism was a provincial national expression opposed to the growth of world revolution. If anyone observed anything like a *bris*, or lighting candles on Friday night, they were reported to the authorities. The only connection I had with Jewish people was by speaking Yiddish with my grandparents; otherwise, I knew nothing about my religion. The same was true of my husband's background. His only connection with the Jewish people was the Yiddish he spoke with his grandparents. It's only when we came to America that we were exposed to Judaism. I really have enjoyed learning about my people and my faith."

"What year did you come to America, Sonja?" Green asked softly.

"My husband and I came to America in the early 1970s.

We were both in our mid-fifties. We were among the first to be allowed to leave. I had an uncle who was very influential in the Communist Party, and he used his influence to permit us to leave."

"Why did you want to leave?"

"Jews didn't have much of a future in Russia. We were told by our hospital directors that our future was limited because, as they put it, of our racial background. Our two boys were harassed often in school by fellow students and even the teachers made disparaging remarks. When we were allowed to leave, we jumped at the opportunity. It meant leaving our families and the friends we had at an advanced age, but it was a chance, and my husband and I felt it was worth it."

"Was your husband a doctor too, Sonja?"

"Yes, he was a neurologist and was very accomplished, but he felt very strongly that we should leave the Soviet Union. He felt that our sons would have a future in America, and that they had very little to look forward to in Russia. He was right."

"How long are you at the center, Sonja?"

"About three years. My husband died five years ago, and sometime after that I felt that I couldn't live alone."

"That must have been some adjustment, coming to America in your mid-fifties, not knowing the language, not being able to practice you profession, having to start all over again."

"Oh, it was, it was, Rabbi. Believe me when I tell you it was a terrible struggle. We knew very little English, and English is such a different language from Russian. We couldn't practice medicine because we didn't have the state license."

"What did you do? How did you support yourself?"

"I got a job as a practical nurse, and my husband got a job as an orderly."

"That must have been quite a come-down from your previous positions."

"Oh, it was, definitely. We had had good positions in a large Moscow hospital and here we were starting on a very low level. But we did okay, as they say in America. We studied for a foreign doctor medical license. I passed after three years, but my husband just couldn't get to know the language well enough."

"That must have depressed him."

"It did. He had a lot of – how do you say it – psychological problems as a result, but he was a good man and we were very attached to each other. It was – how do you say it – wise to leave the Soviet Union when we did. There's been so much trouble there over the last twenty years; nobody knows what the next day will bring. We were extremely fortunate to get out when we did."

"Sonja," Green said glancing at his watch, "it's been nice talking to you. We'll see you at services this Shabbos, okay?"

Green had only peripheral contact with the Soviet regime, and it wasn't pleasant. During the campaign in the '70s to force a very reluctant Soviet government to allow Jews to leave Russia, he went to the New Jersey Cultural Center with members of his community to publicly protest the appearance of the Leningrad Ballet. It was hoped that the demonstration would bring attention to the plight of Soviet Jewry. The group sat quietly waiting for the Ballet's manager to speak to them. The manager came in and asked, "*Immizer fun aich rett Yiddish?*" – Yiddish for "Does anyone here speak Yiddish?" Green nearly fell off his chair. Someone who looked so typically Slavic/Russian was Jewish, and was actually speaking Yiddish to the group! Since Green's Yiddish was quite good, he indicated to the manager, named Morgenstern, what their concerns were. Morgenstern suggested that as the spokesman, Green bring a letter relating their concerns and he would present it to the Soviet Minister of Cultural Affairs. "I'll be glad to do it," Green said, although he thought to himself, *this is not going to go very far at all.*

He brought the letter the next day. He presented it to Morgenstern. They were alone in Morgenstern's hotel room. Morgenstern thanked him for bringing it. He asked Morgenstern, in Yiddish, "What is the situation of the Jews in Russia today?"

Morgenstern looked around surreptitiously and said in Yiddish, "It's not fitting that they should see us alone in one room, you're not a child and you understand what I mean.

"But tell me," Morgenstern continued in Yiddish, "when is Yom Kippur? I want to observe it this year." Green gave him the information, shook hands with him, and left his room choked up. The man was 4,300 miles away from Leningrad . . . and yet he was afraid in New Jersey that someone in his ballet group would report him to the authorities for talking to a Jew.

Another incident was equally painful. Green's grandparents had left Kiev in the 1920s, and settled with his mother, their only child, in Brooklyn. His grandmother's brother and his family had stayed behind in the Ukraine. Contact between the two families was sporadic and inconsistent. His grandparents periodically sent food packages to their family in the Ukraine. Once they received a letter from Clara, his grandmother's sister-in-law, which said the following:

Conditions here in Russia are very good. We have enough of everything. We socialize with family and we often bake and cook together. Sometimes, by chance, I don't measure out enough flour, but fortunately my sister-in-law, who lives two blocks away, comes over with a little more so that we can cook and bake together.

His grandparents knew, of course, that the contents of the letter were false. The only sister-in-law that Clara had was Green's grandmother, who lived in Brooklyn. Obviously, Clara and her family didn't have enough flour and other food to maintain themselves adequately. Due to Soviet censorship, she veiled her plea for more packages.

During the thaw in the Cold War, his grandmother's niece, who lived in Kiev, was permitted to visit her in the U.S. The niece occupied a very prominent position in the medical profession in the Ukraine. She met Green's entire family and was graciously received. Prior to taking leave of them, she asked the family to gather for a photo, which she would take back to the Soviet Union and show to her family. She asked the men in Green's family, who were Orthodox Jews, to take off their yarmulkes for the photograph. Green understood that she was afraid that if by some chance someone in Soviet governmental authority would see that her family in the U.S. practiced Judaism, her position in the Soviet Union would be imperiled.

He then recognized the courageous step that his grandparents had taken to come to America in the 1920s. They came to provide their grandchildren with a life different in every aspect from those who remained in Russia. Their immigration quite legitimately could be termed another Exodus from "bondage to freedom, and from darkness to a great light."

Israel Birnbaum was the resident in Room 205. He was short and very thin. His hands shook perceptively. He was highly intelligent, and Green enjoyed speaking to him. His understanding of current events was keen and incisive. Stamped on his forearm were the numbers signifying suffering, humiliation, pain, and loss. As Birnbaum put it, "All came courtesy of Mr. Hitler's hospitality at Auschwitz." From age fifteen to nineteen he was just a number, a victim subject to the whims of his odious captors. He lost his entire family and most of his friends in the Holocaust.

He had been born into a prosperous family. His family had owned a very large hardware store in the city of Rovno, in Poland. Rovno had been an intensive center of Jewish culture, learning, and Zionism. The Jewish community there consisted of 5,000 families. When the Nazis entered Rovno, they expropriated all Jewish property, including the Birnbaums' family hardware business. In short order, they established a ghetto primarily for children, the infirm, and seniors. Most of Birnbaum's family was incarcerated in the ghetto. Since he was young and strong, Birnbaum was allowed to leave the ghetto at certain times to work for the Nazis in the city. He was able to smuggle some foodstuffs into the ghetto by hiding them under his shirt and pants.

One day when he returned to the ghetto area, he found it completely empty. There was no sound and no answer. He frantically searched everywhere. His youthful voice cried out, "Momma, Abba, Uncle Hershel, brother Shmuel, Tante Feige!" Where had everyone gone? He found out from a gentile friend that the ghetto had been completely evacuated that morning. The ghetto population had been packed into the railroad cars and taken away.

Birnbaum feared the worst. He was enveloped by panic. Later he was to discover the bitter and devastating truth. His family had been taken, along with hundreds of others, to a site sixty kilometers away, and they were all murdered. Yesterday he had been a member of a warm and close-knit family. He had been a son, brother, nephew, and friend.

Today he was bereft of everything. He was an orphan in a monstrous world which, for the most part, showed no kindness, compassion or consideration for him and his people. He observed the *yahrzeit* for his entire family on the Tenth of Tevet, a traditional fast day marking the date that the Romans penetrated the wall of Jerusalem, which enabled them to eventually destroy the Temple. He felt that the destruction of the Rovno ghetto marked the beginning of the Holocaust, the most evil event in Jewish and human history. Consequently, he felt that there was a kind of symmetry between the beginning of the destruction of the Temple and his own personal tragedy, and he utilized the Tenth of Tevet to mark it.

Somehow, with the help of Righteous Gentiles, he survived the war. When he reached the U.S. in 1948, he was alone in the world – completely alone – at the age of nineteen. He got a job with a distant cousin in the so-called "*shmatte* (apparel) business." Eventually he started his own business, and did very well. On one occasion, he told Green, "*Ich hab gemacht zeir a shayn leben*" – "I made a very good living."

Birnbaum married Esther Berman, also a survivor, who worked in the garment industry with him. They had two sons, who were very accomplished. Birnbaum told Rabbi Green sadly, "Esther died three years ago and under the circumstances I decided to move to the Malamud Complex."

Green thought the number seared into Birnbaum's forearm added up to an aggregate of shame for the entire Western world. Any illusions about humanity's basic goodness
and decency were totally shattered during the Nazi regime.
It became painfully clear that humankind was capable of
perpetrating not only acts of evil but acts of absolute evil.
Christianity's claim that it is a religion of love was put to the
test, a test it abjectly failed. The Holocaust, after all, took
place in Christian Europe.

In 1933, the Holy See signed a concordat with Hitler that
helped put a seal of approval on Hitler's murderous regime.
The Muslim world also participated in the cruel murder of
six million innocents. The Mufti of Jerusalem at that time,
Haj Muhammad Amin al-Husseini, joined forces with Hitler
in his monstrously evil plan to exterminate the Jews, and
many Arab leaders were pro-Nazi.

The liberal Western democracies also participated in the
abominable criminality of the Holocaust. France handed
over 75,000 Jews to be slaughtered by the Nazis. England
sealed the docks of Palestine, not permitting Jews to enter
during that period of persecution and destruction. Eastern
European countries – Poland and Ukraine, the Baltic States,
Croatia and others – engaged in terrible incidents of acts of
mass murder perpetrated by the Nazis, in which local pop-
ulations often participated avidly. Even the greatest liberal
democracy, the U.S., refused to change its antiquated and
cruel quota system, and virtually no Jews were permitted to
come into the country just before and during the war.

FDR was an icon to American Jews – it would not be
inaccurate to say that many of them worshipped him. He
proved, however, to be an idol with clay feet, and showed

great indifference to the plight of European Jewry. During the Holocaust, the Jews were alone, powerless, and deserted.

Birnbaum, Green thought, *was not a survivor – that was too minimal a term. He was a hero! In his own way, he had triumphed over the Nazis and Hitler. He had established a family, had been successful in business, and participated in his Jewish community. He was a paradigm of his first name "Israel." He had grappled with humanity and with God and had triumphed.*

Green often thought of the tremendous heroism that so many people display in their lives. They are unheralded. Except for their families, few know the tribulations they experienced. The residents at Malamud exemplified this. Weiner without a father for nine very crucial years of his life. Grossman coming to the South from Lithuania, a greenhorn, then going north to attend NYU. Mrs. Rosenblatt losing both parents by the age of eleven, and then her daughter in her middle age. Sonja coming in her fifties to a new society so different from the one in which she had previously lived. Danzig supporting his mother and trying to be helpful in so many different ways. Birnbaum living a hellish existence in his youth with so many adjustments to make.

I'm sure, Green thought, *many residents of the home have similar stories. When you think of what was happening around them while they were growing up: World War I, the Depression, World War II, the Holocaust in which many residents lost many of their family in Europe, raising a family in times of such turmoil and change. None of them had a life of comfort and contentment. No wonder some are depressed and nervous, and some have difficulty relating to others. Life has been tough and, in some cases, mean and unfair to them. Yet they all had a certain dignity, a sense of having done the best they could under the circumstances they faced. What else could anyone ask of them? They all had remained decent and kindly human beings. Maybe that's the real test of success in life.*

Green realized that experiences shape a person's character – how he responds to misfortune, or for that matter, good fortune. Does he become mean and indifferent? Or does he integrate these unfortunate experiences and become a smarter, wiser, and perhaps tougher person? Does he retain an essential decency about himself and how he relates to others?

There were tremendous life lessons to learn at the geriatric center and, as experience added to experience, he began to appreciate the environment. It was helping him to become a wiser person, one who appreciated life more. He could see that his life, like everyone's, was not endless. He had to do the best he could with the moments that he had.

*

ONE OF GREEN'S DUTIES was to visit the Morgan Hospital in Bucks County Pennsylvania, where there were always many Jewish patients. There were many transplanted New Yorkers living in the area which the hospital served. Since he was originally from Brooklyn, there were many opportunities to share nostalgic memories with the patients. He often could see the patients relaxing during these conversations, smiling as meaningful memories were revisited. If they would agree, he would recite the *Mi SheBerach* – a prayer for their recovery. Invariably the patient was grateful and expressed appreciation for the visit.

On occasion, the visit consisted of saying a quick hello

to the patient, who was highly medicated and in great pain. Understandably, the patient's response was minimal. Yet he always left his card – a gesture that demonstrated the concern of the Philadelphia Jewish community for the patient.

The contemporary world of medicine was impersonal and structured on the business model. The patient was jabbed, stuck, pricked, measured – virtually every one of his orifices was invaded; he was sent from X-ray to MRI or PET scan like a ping pong ball. The staff was overworked, stressed out, burnt out. Where there should have been ten nurses on the floor, there were six. Because of capitation payments, the doctors usually spent four to five minutes with a patient, and then on to the next one. One doctor told him of a practice that saw 125 patients a day in order to remain financially viable. Thus, the touch of humanity he provided was absolutely vital.

The business model led to low morale of the medical staff, while the salaries of the hospital administrators were extremely high. There were layers upon layers of bureaucracy. Associate administrators piled on associate administrators, all receiving very fine wages.

Recently, the position of "Hospitalist" was established. A doctor who was not any individual patient's doctor, but was employed by the hospital, saw many of the patients. This was clearly a disaster waiting to happen. How well did the hospitalist know the patient? The hospitalist had little knowledge of the patient's health background and virtually no knowledge at all of his family situation. The encounter was brief . . . and then on to the next patient. As with most things in the modern hospital, human contact was kept to a minimum.

In an institution as complex as the modern hospital, medications could be confused and test results shared mistakenly with the wrong family. This situation even happened to Green. As a patient himself once, he was supposed to get a particular antibiotic. The nurse was about to administer it when his wife Sara noticed that it was the wrong medication. The nurse insisted that it was the right one. Finally, after much insistence on Sara's part, the nurse consented to check. The medication in fact was for another Green on the same floor.

A patient must have an advocate! Green often thought to himself. He constantly heard complaints from patients in great pain that they had been ringing for a nurse for half an hour, and no one had come in to help them. Generally, the health care delivery situation in contemporary America was awful. Over 40 million Americans had no medical insurance. When they needed medical care, they had to go to the emergency room. And if a patient had a difficult heart or kidney condition, how much could the emergency physician do except to stabilize him?

Green recognized that some hospitals try to provide high-level health care as well as employee recognition. Many hospitals display warm notes from patients and their families, thanking the nursing staff and other employees for their kind and effective professional skills. But as long as the bottom line was the primary goal of the hospital, and health care was considered an industry, limitations existed that could imperil patients' health and fray the tempers of all members of the staff.

When he needed support and encouragement, Green turned to three poignant letters. They described the pain of the hospital experience and expressed the vulnerability that nearly overwhelmed them, as well as their appreciation of his intervention.

Dear Rabbi Green,

In May I met you when my mother was having heart surgery. I took your card with the intention of writing you immediately to thank you for being so wonderful to my family and me. Of course, I delayed and forgot about it. As I was cleaning out my purse this morning, I found your card.

My whole family was very frustrated because we were so worried about Mother and couldn't talk to a doctor. You came into the hospitality room and sat and talked with all of us for some time and then you came up to C.C.U. to check in on Mother several times. Thank you. I cannot impress upon you how important it was to me to know that someone cared.

I hope all is well for you.

Sincerely,
Mary Burns

P.S.   Mother is doing great!

Dear Rabbi Green,

I know you hear over and over in your work how people appreciate your services. However, none of them could be as genuine as my "thank you" for the supportive comfort you gave me this morning. Being alone in this world, going through a trying experience, is difficult! However, having a messenger of God at one's side does lighten the burden. The results of the cath were satisfactory and it has been decided to have Bill go along a conservative therapeutic route.

May you and your family enjoy a healthy and happy holiday season.

Most sincerely,
Roberta Evans, M.D.

Dear Rabbi Green,

I just want to let you know how much I appreciated your words of comfort and support to my family in the moments before, during, and after my father's death. It was nice to have such a caring person with us as we were experiencing the difficult parts of life.

You have a gentle and sensitive approach; my wife commented that although she did not feel like getting into a deep discussion at the time, she was comforted to know you were there, showing your concern for our loss by your very presence. Somehow the horror of the moment and unfamiliarity with the hospital and medical procedures were eased somewhat by your thoughtful gestures, such as cold water for my grieving mother.

Thank you again, Rabbi Green, for the kindness and comfort shown to my family at our time of great loss. God bless you and your work.

Respectfully,
Bradley Johnson II

Occasionally, when he looked at these letters, he was reminded of the statement of the Hebrew sages in Tractate *Shabbos* 127a: "Visiting the sick is an observance whose fruits a person enjoys in this world but whose principal remains intact for him in the World to Come." To support people when they are ill, alone, and isolated is to participate in that which is eternal and everlasting.

*

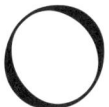NCE A MONTH, GREEN visited the maximum security Greenwood Reformatory, just outside of Philadelphia. It was one of the oldest prisons in

the country. Everything about it appeared stark and sinister. The prison walls were 25-feet high with guards posted in their tower sites fully armed. At night, search lights swept the entire prison area, emphasizing the darkness even more. The inmates had no privacy. The bars on the cells were open so that everything could be seen from the outside – the toilet, the sink, the cot, everything! The few phone calls the inmates were allowed to make per month were monitored. The letters received were censored. The visits from family were severely limited and were listened to by the guards, who would often taunt the inmates: "You thought you were such a big deal city slicker!" Or, they would say, "The college degree you got really got you places, big shot!"

The prison inmates were male. Some of the wards were guarded by female guards. Some of the inmates deeply resented being guarded by females. There was always the danger of rape. He vividly remembered how one of the inmates came into his office in a state of great agitation. "Rabbi Green," he said in a quiet anxious tone, "you must get me out of the section I'm in. I'm afraid I'm going to be raped." Green got on the phone immediately with the assistant superintendent, and the inmate's domicile was changed immediately.

When Green began his duties at the prison, the drug scene was in full force. The Jewish inmates, like everyone else, had been selling, buying, and committing hold-ups to get the money to buy drugs. They were mostly from middle-class backgrounds. One had attended an Ivy League university. All were high school graduates and very bright young people. They were attracted by the easy money they thought drugs would bring, or had become addicted to drugs and would do anything to get them.

Most of the parents came every Visitors Day. They would break into tears when speaking of their son. The jarring constant refrain was how pained they were to have a son who could steal, commit holdups, threaten, and assault others. These acts were against everything they stood for, and in opposition to how they had raised their son. They all had a deep sense of having been betrayed. While they were not religiously observant, there was in all of them a sense of *shanda* – shame, embarrassment, humiliation, and pain.

Not all Jewish inmates were incarcerated because of drugs. A very egregious case which depressed Green every time he thought of it was that of Herb Derman. Herb was a tall, good-looking young man who had molested a young girl. He was in a special isolation unit under heavy security. There was an "honor code" amongst the inmates – anyone guilty of molestation was in serious danger of being killed by the other inmates. The authorities took special precautions to prevent that from happening, and segregated these inmates.

Herb came from a very affluent family that was well-known and highly regarded in their community. His mother came to speak to Green every visiting day. She was a tall, elegant, and attractive woman. She was overwhelmed by the tragedy that had overtaken her family. "Rabbi Green," she said, "you're the only one who cares for him. I often think that his life is in danger on a daily basis. My husband and I jump every time the phone rings at home." She began crying.

"You know, Rabbi Green," she said, tears pouring down her cheeks, "driving here this morning, I thought to myself,

I wish I had lost him when I was carrying him." She took out her handkerchief and sobbed with great intensity.

There was silence . . . a silence so foreboding that it threatened to envelop both of them in despair. In this inhumane place, he felt that he was the only anchor of human concern and compassion.

At the nursing home, he was an anchor amidst inevitable decline. At the prison, however, the possibility of rehabilitation and redemption remained. This was expressed to him in a letter from the Ivy League graduate after his release from Greenwood.

Dear Rabbi Green,

I am realizing only now how fruitful my experience was, and is, in knowing you. Even now, though, I cannot tell you what exactly you were for me and to me. At times you were a listener where there was no other. On other occasions, you were my tie with the outer world; but these are only tangible manifestations of your life to me, and to the other boys. Far more, there exists another quality about you which brings the comfort, the peace that one needs so badly in that otherwise God-forsaken land. I know that it is not always easy for you to become involved, as you necessarily must, with the fellows, in order to produce the effects of this quality you possess. However, I can tell you now – now that the nightmare is over for me – that not doing so renders you ineffective in your capacity as a spiritual leader and equally ineffective as a man. There are very few men as fortunate as you who possess both the capacity and the opportunity to affect a fellow human as much and as positively as you can.

I wonder if you are as aware of this responsibility, which is also a blessing, as I am (having been to the other side, so to speak).

And now, even more than before (since I can see your life against the vast panorama of the multitude of relatively "nothing" lives I see around here in the "real world"), I am beginning to fully appreciate what a few men like yourself can mean to a lost, lonely boy – maybe even a lost, lonely world. Oh, make no mistake about it, you can't do very much; the world will go on as it has, and as it must. But maybe there will be just one or two lives you will touch, and for the possibility of that, you must always try. I can only speak for myself, yet I can say that for me you made a crucial difference. Perhaps for others, you will have to do more – if necessary, then do it! Because that is all you have – truly that is all we all have. But that is the difference, and will always be to me. God exists in the process of gleaning a hint of another human soul.

I hope I will be hearing from you soon. Please give my regards to everyone. My best wishes to your wife and daughters for a healthy year. Please try to write soon, Rabbi, as I am looking forward to hearing from you.

Sincerely,
Bill Ruben

*

ALBERT CAMUS SPOKE OF life as being "absurd." Thousands of years before Camus, the author of *Ecclesiastes* had said something quite similar: "Vanity of vanities, all is vanity. What profits a man with all his labor when he labors under the sun?" It is true that life often is unjust, frustrating, and depressing. At times, it appears to be purposeless and lacking in meaning, and filled with empty routine. Green was convinced that the way to overcome this numbing nihilism was through giving to others. In that way, one expands the circumference of his existence, and his essence achieves greater depth.

Camus leaves us with a devastating sense of life's impermanence and helplessness. The author of *Ecclesiastes* was aware of these conditions, too. At the end of his classic work, he proposed an answer. He wrote, "At the end of the matter, all having been heard, fear God and keep His commandments, for this is the whole person."

Green reflected: *If you want to overcome the despair, the impermanence, and seeming purposelessness of life, attach yourself to the eternal and the transcendent.*

If we consider these as sacred responsibilities and not just choices, then we do have purpose, meaning, and direction. Our existence continually takes on more and more nuances, shadings, and essences, and we are not rudderless in the vast and often tempest-tossed sea of life.

בזה אני מברך על המוגמר
"הודו לה׳ כי טוב כי לעולם חסדו"

ABOUT THE AUTHOR

Rabbi SIDNEY GOLDSTEIN is a graduate of Yeshiva University from which he received a B.A. in History. He was granted *Smicha* (rabbinic ordination) by the Rabbi Isaac Elchanan Theological Seminary of YU. He later earned a Ph.D. in Rabbinic Literature from the Bernard Revel Graduate School of YU.

Rabbi Goldstein authored the book *Suicide in Rabbinic Literature*. He also wrote many articles in rabbinic journals. He helped found and is a former President of the National Association of Jewish Chaplains.

Rabbi Goldstein has held pulpits in Elmira, N.Y., and Asbury Park, N.J. He was the Director of Chaplaincy at the Albert Einstein Medical Center in Philadelphia, PA, and the Jewish Family Service of South Palm Beach County, Boca Raton, FL. He has taught at Brookdale Community College, Monmouth University, and was a visiting professor of Religion and Philosophy at Palm Beach State College.

He and his wife Marilyn are thankful to reside in Jerusalem, Israel. They are blessed with two daughters, grandchildren, and great-grandchildren.